A Manual Cardiac Surgical Intensive Care

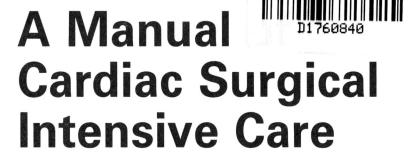

A Manual of Cardiac Surgical Intensive Care

Russell Millner and John Pepper

Department of Cardiac Surgery, St George's Hospital
London

Edward Arnold
A division of Hodder & Stoughton
LONDON   MELBOURNE   AUCKLAND

© 1990 Russell Millner and John Pepper

First published in Great Britain 1990

British Library Cataloguing in Publication Data

Millner, Russell
  A manual of cardiac surgical intensive care.
  1. Man. Heart. Surgery. Postperative intensive care
  I. Title II. Pepper, John
  617.412028

  ISBN 0–340–52855–9

Whilst the advice and information in this book is believed to be
true and accurate at the date of going to press, neither the author
nor the publisher can accept any legal responsibility or liability
for any errors or omissions that may be made. In particular (but
without limiting the generality of the preceding disclaimer) every
effort has been made to check drug dosages; however, it is still
possible that errors have been missed. Furthermore, dosage
schedules are being continually revised and new side effects
recognised. For these reasons the reader is strongly urged to
consult the drug companies' printed instructions before
administering any of the drugs recommended in this book.

Typeset in 9/10 pt Times by TecSet, Wallington, Surrey
Printed by St Edmundsbury Press Ltd, Bury St Edmunds,
Suffolk, and bound by W. H. Ware & Sons Ltd, Avon, for
Edward Arnold, a division of Hodder and Stoughton Limited, Mill
Road, Dunton Green, Sevenoaks, Kent TN13 2YA

Preface

As the volume of cardiac surgery increases, many more junior staff, both medical and nursing, will be exposed to its complexities. There is a requirement for easily available and uncomplicated information and advice on the wide range of problems that may be met in the cardiac surgical patient. It is important for the safety of the patient and the peace of mind of junior staff that they should have a working knowledge of the management of the more common emergencies.

This book is designed to be an easily available collection of background material relevant to the subject, flow charts on management decisions, and finally a ready source of drug and physiological data.

Although it is designed to be a practical guide for use by doctors who are working on a post-operative cardiac surgical intensive care unit, it should also be a convenient source of quick reference for nurses on the unit. In particular it should help those who are undertaking post-registration cardiac nursing courses.

No handbook must ever detract from the overriding principle of 'get help if you are in trouble'; however, this one provides front-line pathways for the treatment of the acute problems arising in and around the cardiac surgical intensive care unit.

The book is structured in three parts; first, background to the specialty, including anatomy, physiology and pharmacology. The second part contains the problem-orientated management algorithms. The third and final part contains list of drug doses, inotropic infusion tables, conversion factors and physiological data.

We would like to thank Ms Pauline Stokes, RGN, and Dr Peter Sutton for their help with specific points. Any errors or omissions are ours.

Whilst every effort has been made to check the accuracy of the drug and physiological data, it must remain the prescriber's responsibility to ensure that a drug dose is correct before it is given.

Contents

Part 1

The aim of this part of the handbook is to provide background anatomy, physiology and pharmacology. Also included are descriptions of the more commonly used invasive techniques which are available for use in the intensive care setting.

1

The history of cardiac surgery

The development of cardiac surgery runs in parallel with much of the development of modern surgery. This in turn is dependent upon progress in allied fields.

In 1813 Legallois presented the concept of a paracorporeal circulation. In 1882 Von Schroder proposed the concept of the bubble oxygenator. Von Frey in 1885 and Gruber and Jacobi in 1890 and later on De Bakey in 1934, Lindberg and Alexis Carrell all proposed varying types of pumps and bypass mechanisms for extracorporeal perfusion. Gibbon in 1936 started research work in cats but it was not until Dennis in 1951 and, again, Gibbon in 1954 that clinically effective bypass pumps became available.

During the same period Landsteiner in 1900 discovered the blood groups and in 1918 Howell and Holt discovered Heparin. These two discoveries were of crucial importance for the future development of cardiac surgery.

Lillehei in 1955 began using cardiopulmonary bypass in infants using a simple pump and one of the parents as the oxygenator. Mechanical oxygenators were developed by Crafoord and Andersen in 1948. In the decade that followed, many others including Melrose in 1953 described other experimental oxygenator systems. Kirklin in 1955 was one of the first to undertake cardiac surgery using full cardiopulmonary bypass; he used a version of the equipment described by Gibbon in 1951.

In the early years, the major problem after cardiac surgery was the persistence of low cardiac output in the post-operative period. At first surgeons blamed the pre-operative state of the patient. It was Najafai in 1968 who showed that many patients were suffering large sub-endocardial infarcts during surgery. Together with the massive explosion in surgery for coronary artery disease this forced surgeons into looking more carefully at techniques of myocardial preservation.

Over the years as cardiac surgery has developed, many forms of myocardial preservation have been developed. Lewis and Taufic in 1953 performed intracardiac repairs under hypothermia. Sealy in 1957 and Drew and Anderson in 1958 used the combination of extracorporeal circulation and profound hypothermia.

Whilst Melrose in 1955 put forward the concept of chemical arrest of the heart with large concentrations of potassium, Helmsworth subsequently in 1959 observed direct myocardial injury by potassium citrate and the early attempts at cardioplegia were largely abandoned. Shumway in 1959 popularised intermittent ischaemic arrest with topical cardiac hypothermia from which the technique of cross-clamp fibrillation was eventually developed.

In the meantime, Bretschneider and Kirsch had continued to study cardioplegia as had Hearse. These are cold solutions that are injected into the aortic root or the coronary arteries directly, leading to a rapid electromechanical arrest in diastole. Part of the preservation arises from this arrest and part from ensuring that the heart is kept cool with both topical cooling of the heart and also systemic cooling of the patient. Sundergaard in 1975 published the clinical use of Bretschneider's solution. Braimbridge in 1977 described the use of the St Thomas' cardioplegic solution which had been developed by Hearse. Whilst these are both crystalloid solutions, they differ in that the Bretschneider solution is predominately an intracellular concentration of ions whilst that of Hearse is extracellular. Buckberg in 1978 described cold blood as a carrier for his cardioplegic solutions and undoubtedly the final story is not yet written.

A high proportion of modern cardiac surgery is concerned with myocardial revascularisation, its success being based on a detailed knowledge of each individual patient's coronary anatomy and on a meticulous surgical technique. Judkin and Mason Sones in the early 1960s developed techniques of coronary arteriography. Before that in 1946 Vineberg introduced the technique of implanting the freely bleeding ends of the internal thoracic (mammary) arteries directly into the myocardium. Direct coronary artery bypass surgery with saphenous vein was first reported by Sabiston in 1962 though it was Favoloro who popularised the technique. In 1968 Green reported the use of internal thoracic (mammary) artery for coronary artery bypass surgery.

Open valvular heart surgery started in the mid-1950s with aortic valvulotomy and removal of calcium deposits. It became apparent that this alone was not always enough and partial prosthetic valve replacement with replacement of diseased leaflets was tried. Results were still not good and in 1958 both Muller and Lillehei replaced the entire aortic valve with a prosthesis. Hufnagel in 1951 had inserted a ball-valve prosthesis in the descending thoracic aorta for the palliation of patients with severe aortic incompetence before the era of cardiopulmonary bypass. The development of Starr's ball-in-cage prosthesis was a very major step forward in the early 1960s and since then there have been many different mechanical and tissue valves developed.

The mechanical valves currently in use fall into three major groups. The ball-in-cage valves as exemplified by the Starr–Edwards valve, the tilting disc valves such as the Bjork–Shiley, and the bileaflet design such as the St Jude or Carbomedics designs (Fig. 1.1).

Fig. 1.1 (a) Starr-Edwards; (b) Bjork-Shiley; (c) St Jude.

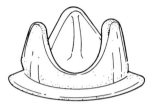

Fig. 1.2 Carpentier-Edwards type.

The tissue valves fall into three main groups. First the xenograft (pig) aortic valves mounted in a stent, the xenograft pericardium (bovine) fashioned into cusps and then mounted in stents. Examples of the first group include the Carpentier–Edwards (Fig. 1.2), Medtronic Intac and Wessex Valves and of the second group the Bioflo valve that is in current use and the Ionescu–Shiley valve that has now been withdrawn. The third main group is the Homograft aortic valve whose use has been popularised by Ross in England and Barratt-Boyes in New Zealand.

2
Autonomic physiology

Control of vegetative function lies in the autonomic nervous system. This comprises two complementary and frequently opposing systems.

The outflow from the central nervous system lies in the sympathetic and parasympathetic divisions of the autonomic nervous system. There is an anatomical and physiological separation into the two divisions (Fig. 2.1).

Both divisions have pre-ganglionic and post-ganglionic fibres and then an effector organ. The differences lie in the relative lengths of the pre- and post-ganglionic fibres, and the nature of the transmitter substances at the various ganglia.

The sympathetic system has short pre-ganglionic fibres, arriving in the para-vertebral ganglia via the white rami communicantes where they end on the cell bodies of the post-synaptic fibres. These in turn are distributed via the grey rami communicantes to their effector organis. Whilst the sympathetic outflow is from the first thoracic to third lumbar ventral roots of the spinal cord, the parasympathetic outflow is in two separate components; first there is a cranial nerve outflow in the 3rd, 7th, 9th, 10th cranial nerves, and second there is a sacral outflow in the 2nd, 3rd, and 4th sacral nerves. (See Fig. 2.2).

Unlike the sympathetic system, the pre-ganglionic fibres in the para-sympathetic system are long with short post-ganglionic fibres, which often lie within the effector organs

The main autonomic neurotransmitters are acetylcholine and noradrenaline. All pre-ganglionic fibres are cholinergic, as are the post-ganglionic parasympathetic fibres, together with the post-ganglionic sympathetic vasodilator fibres to skeletal muscle blood vessels.

The post-ganglionic synapses at the effector organs in the noradrenergic sympathetic system can be divided into two groups on the basis of the behaviour of the receptors to different agents.

These two subtypes of receptors are described as alpha and beta. In turn each of these subgroups is divided into two further groups; alpha 1, alpha 2 and beta 1, beta 2.

Alpha receptors are more sensitive to adrenaline and noradrenaline than to isoprenaline. Both beta 1 and beta 2 receptors are very sensitive to isoprenaline. Beta 2 are more sensitive to adrenaline than noradrenaline,

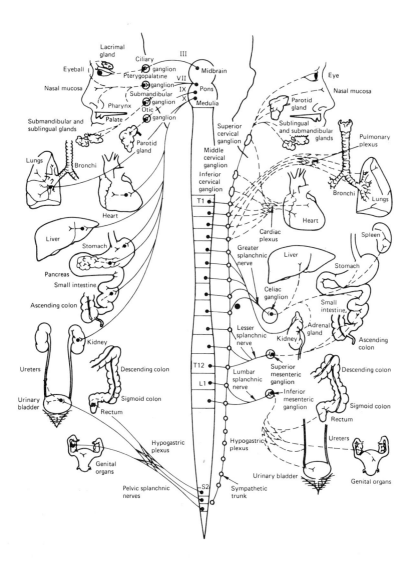

Fig. 2.1 Structure of the autonomic nervous system. The parasympathetic division is shown only on the left side of the figure and the sympathetic division is shown only on the right side.

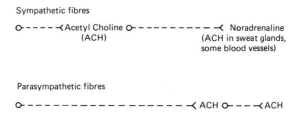

Sympathetic fibres

O- - - - -≺Acetyl Choline O- - - - - - - - - - ≺ Noradrenaline
(ACH)   (ACH in sweat glands,
                                   some blood vessels)

Parasympathetic fibres

O- - - - - - - - - - - - - - - - - - ≺ ACH O- - - ≺ ACH

Fig. 2.2   The sympathetic system.

	Adrenaline	Noradrenaline	Isoprenaline
alpha	+ + +	+ + +	+
beta 1	+ +	+ +	+ + +
beta 2	+ +	+	+ + +

Fig. 2.3   Schematic representation of relative sensitivities.

whilst beta 1 are equally sensitive to adrenaline and noradrenaline. (See Fig. 2.3).

In the heart, the predominant noradrenergic receptor is the beta 1 type. In the conduction system, beta 1 stimulation of the sino-atrial node increases the frequency of depolarisation, and in the atrio-ventricular node and Bundle of His it increases the conduction velocity. In both the atria and ventricles it increases both contractility and conduction velocity. Cholinergic [parasympathetic] stimulation, mediated through the vagus [10th cranial] nerve has opposite effects, reducing the rate of sino-atrial node depolarization, and slowing the conduction through the atrio-ventricular node and Bundle of His, though not reducing contractility.

In the vascular system, including coronary, renal, pulmonary and muscle beds, parasympathetic cholinergic stimulation and sympathetic noradrenergic beta 2 stimulation both cause vasodilation. However, sympathetic noradrenergic alpha stimulation causes vasoconstriction.

In the lungs parasympathetic cholinergic stimulation causes broncho-constriction together with increased production of bronchial secretions. Adrenergic beta 2 stimulation causes bronchodilation.

In the kidney, renal blood flow is increased by specific dopaminergic receptors. This effect is independent of cholinergic or beta 2 induced renal artery vasodilation (*see* Fig. 2.4).

In the adrenal glands, the medulla can be thought of as a post-ganglionic synapse, secreting adrenaline and noradrenaline directly into the blood stream.

	Alpha	Beta 1	Beta 2	Parasympathetic	Dopaminergic
Heart:	– – – – – –	Increase rate and contractility	– – – – – –	Decrease rate	Increase rate and contractility at higher dose
Lungs:	– – – – – –	– – – – – –	Bronchodilation	Bronchoconstriction	– – – – – –
Vascular:	Constrict	– – – – – –	Dilate	Dilate	Constrict at higher dose
Kidney:	Vasoconstrict	– – – – – –	Vasodilate	Vasodilate	Vasodilate at low dose

Fig. 2.4 Simplified receptor effects.

Control of blood pressure

Reflex control of blood pressure lies in a series of feedback loops. Receptors are found both in the pre-load or venous side of the system including both atria (volume receptors) and also in the after-load or arterial side of the circulation (pressure receptors). The arterial baro-receptors lie in the aortic arch and carotid sinus. (The terms pre- and after-load are derived from isolated cardiac muscle preparations; however, they are useful in understanding the behaviour of the myocardium in vivo.)

Afferent fibres run in the 9th and 10th cranial nerves to the medulla oblongata and produce inhibition of vasoconstriction and activation of vasodilation.

From the brain stem run the pathways that lead to the sympathetic nervous system, with fibres ending on the resistance producing arterioles. As mentioned in the previous section, there are amongst these both vasodilator cholinergic fibres and also noradrenergic vasoconstrictor fibres. There is usually a tonic discharge to the vasoconstrictor fibres, which ensures the maintenance of an adequate blood pressure under normal conditions (Fig. 2.5).

Apart from the neural control, circulating adrenaline, noradrenaline, angiotensin and local metabolic factors contribute to the maintenance of an adequate blood pressure.

Impaired renal blood flow leads to the production of renin, which leads to the activation of angiotensin 1 from angiotensinogen. Angiotensin 1 in turn leads to the production of angiotensin 2, in the lungs, which then stimulates the secretion of aldosterone. In the kidney, aldosterone acts to retain sodium and hence water. This then helps to maintain the extracellular and intravascular fluid volumes (Fig. 2.6).

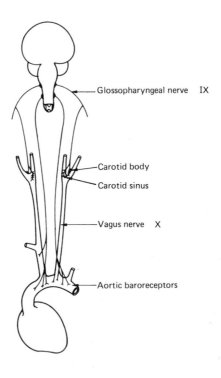

Glossopharyngeal nerve   IX

Carotid body

Carotid sinus

Vagus nerve   X

Aortic baroreceptors

Fig. 2.5   The baroreceptor system.

The baroreceptor mediated reflexes provide short-term, acute control of blood pressure, though as they adapt within 48 h, they do not provide longer-term control. The renal mechanism contributes to longer-term control but not to acute changes in blood pressure.

Current evidence would suggest that stretch receptors in the atria and pulmonary veins respond to distension and hence changes in blood volume by decreasing their rate of firing with decreased stretch. In turn this leads to an increase in anti-diuretic hormone (ADH) release and a decrease in the release of atrial naturetic peptides and consequently sodium retention in the kidney.

Local metabolic factors contribute to the control of the circulation by producing changes in resistance arterioles. Increasing concentrations of

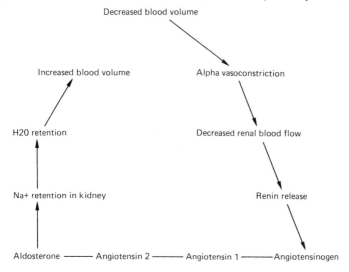

Fig. 2.6

by-products of metabolism dilate the vessels and allow an increase in local blood flow and therefore a decrease in systemic vascular resistance when combined with similar processes elsewhere. Increasing tissue activity or a decrease in regional blood flow leads to the accumulation of ADP and AMP, together with an increase in K^+ and H^+ (a fall in pH). Also there is a rise in local pCO_2 and a fall in pO_2. All these factors will lead to a local vasodilation and an increase in local blood flow, which in turn will tend to reverse their accumulation and therefore complete a homeostatic feedback loop. In clinical terms, this is the phenomenon of reactive hyperaemia (Fig. 2.7).

Heart rate is controlled through similar afferent pathways to those detailed above, noradrenergic sympathetic nerves increase both the rate and force of contraction, as do the circulating catecholamines (though the reflex bradycardia of noradrenaline may manifest as a net effect of a slowing in heart rate). Cholinergic vagal fibres slow the heart.

The best clinical demonstration of these effects is in the state of hypovolaemic shock. The essential changes are of a reduced blood volume, and hence pre-load, reflected in a low CVP. Arterial baroreceptors also receive less stimulation. As a consequence the inhibition of vasoconstriction is reduced and arteriolar constriction ensues. Similarly venoconstriction occurs and this augments the return of blood to the right side of the heart. At the same time, adrenergic stimulation of the heart leads to an increase in both heart rate and contractility. Catecholamines

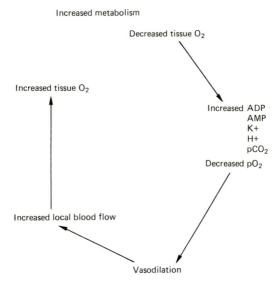

Increased metabolism

Fig. 2.7

are released by the adrenal medulla, as are glucocorticoids and mineraldo-corticoids from the adrenal cortex.

A fall in renal blood flow precipitates the release of Renin and the activation of the renin–angiotensin–aldosterone system. Aldosterone inhibits Na^+ excretion by the kidneys, which in turn will lead to an increase in plasma oncotic pressure and therefore the movement of water across capillary membranes from the extravascular space into the intravascular space. Pituitary release of vasopressin (ADH) inhibits renal excretion of water and this combines with the Na^+ retention to increase the circulating blood volume.

Other adrenergic effects include a reduced skin blood flow together with sweating, which can be measured by a fall in peripheral temperature.

Special circulations

Coronary circulation

5% of the cardiac output at rest passes through the coronary circulation. This is equal to 250 ml/min, and as there is a very high degree of oxygen extraction from this blood, then an increase in myocardial O_2 requirement during exercise can only be met by an increase in coronary blood flow.

Coronary vasodilation is dependent on local factors as described above. It is important to remember that coronary blood flow is phasic depending on the cardiac cycle, the majority of flow to the left ventricle occurring during diastole when the myocardium is relaxed. Therefore the pressure gradient across the myocardium at this time is the major governing factor for coronary blood flow. If the diastolic pressure should fall or the intraventricular pressure (as reflected by the end-diastolic pressure) should rise, then coronary blood flow will tend to fall (Fig. 2.8).

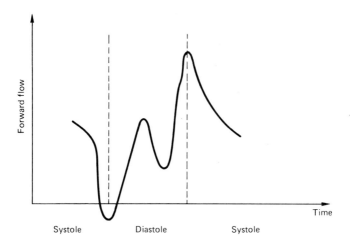

Fig. 2.8 Coronary blood flow.

Pulmonary circulation

The control of the pulmonary circulation lies in both local and systematic factors; there are both alpha adrenergic receptors that cause pulmonary vasoconstriction and also some vagal receptors that lead to mild pulmonary vasodilation. In addition there is also a series of local autoregulatory mechanisms; a fall in alveolar ventilation leads to a decrease in pO_2, which in turn leads to pulmonary vasoconstriction and to both a decrease in pulmonary perfusion and an increase in pulmonary vascular resistance (Fig. 2.9).

In a similar way, a decrease in pulmonary perfusion will lead to an increased alveolar pCO_2 and in turn to bronchoconstriction and a concomitant fall in alveolar ventilation. At the same time a decrease in perfusion is followed by a lessening in surfactant production and a tendency towards alveolar collapse and impaired alveolar ventilation (Fig. 2.10).

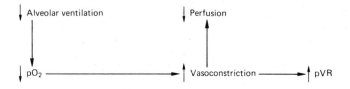

Fig. 2.9

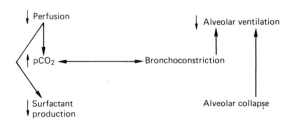

Fig. 2.10

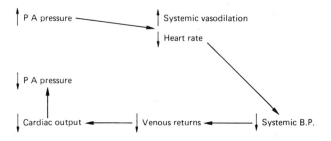

Fig. 2.11

A fall in the blood pH leads to vasoconstriction and increased pulmonary vascular resistance.

There is also a series of acute reflexes associated with the pulmonary artery; an abrupt increase in pulmonary artery pressure is met by a decrease in heart rate and systemic vasodilation. In turn this leads to a fall in systemic blood pressure and a decrease in venous return. From this follows a fall in cardiac output and a return of pulmonary artery pressure to a lower level (Fig. 2.11).

3
Cardiac anatomy and physiology

The heart is simply a pump, though not a simple one. In reality it consists of two separate pumps, the right and left atrio-ventricular complexes, beating in series and in a coordinated manner.

The normal heart consists of two atria, these being low-pressure priming chambers that receive blood from either systemic or pulmonary veins. Each atrium is connected through an atrio-ventricular valve to its appropriate ventricle, that on the right side being the tri-leaflet tricuspid valve and that on the left the bi-leaflet mitral valve. Each ventricle ejects blood through a usually tricuspid valve, the pulmonary on the right and aortic valve on the left. Above the aortic valve are three dilations in the root of the aorta each corresponding to a cusp of the valve. These are the sinuses of Valsava, and from two of these arise the coronary arteries.

The left main-stem artery arises from the posterior sinus and runs behind the pulmonary artery; within 1–2 cm it divides into two branches: the left anterior descending which runs across the front of the heart in the groove between right and left ventricles, and the circumflex coronary artery which runs back in the groove between left atrium and left ventricle. Both these arteries give off a number of significant branches. The right coronary artery arises from the anterior sinus and turns to the right passing under the right atrial appendage to run down in the right atrio-ventricular groove until it gives off the posterior descending branch which lies in the posterior groove between left and right ventricles.

Cardiac muscle shows a series of fundamental properties that set it apart from other types of muscle, the most important being the ability of pacemaker regions to undergo spontaneous depolarisation and produce rhythmic contraction. It behaves as a slow twitch muscle with consequent resistance to fatigue. Its inability to undergo further depolarisation during most of its action potential produces its resistance to tetany.

Electrical excitation starts in the spontaneously depolarising sino-atrial node, situated at the junction of superior vena cava and right atrium. The impulse is transmitted through the atrial musculature to the atrio-ventricular node, which is located in the right side of the posterior portion of the atrial septum close to the coronary sinus.

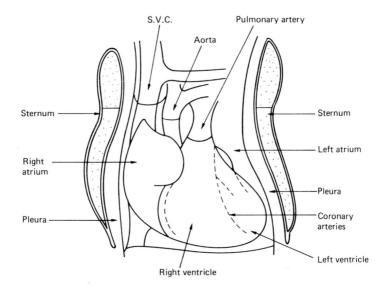

Fig. 3.1 The heart as seen at median sternotomy

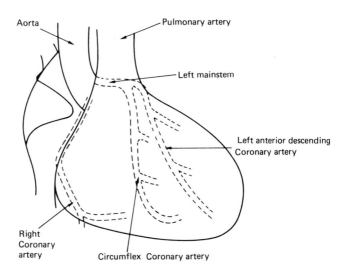

Fig. 3.2 Diagrammatic projection of a coronary arteriogram onto an outline of the heart

The atrio-ventricular node slows the impulse before passing it into the Bundle of His, which disseminates the impulse to the ventricular masses. The Bundle of His crosses the atrio-ventricular ring and then runs along the inferior portion of the membranous septum. Continuing along the upper portion of the muscular septum, it divides into the right and left branches. The right branch passes down the right side of the septum, mostly to the anterior wall of the right ventricle. The left branch passes down the left side of the muscular interventricular septum, dividing into anterior and posterior hemi fascicles, supplying the left ventricular muscle mass.

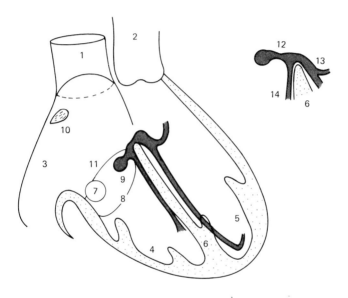

Fig. 3.3 Anatomy of the conduction system

1	SVC	2	Aorta
3	Right atrium	4	Right ventricle
5	Left ventricle	6	Ventricular septum
7	Coronary sinus	8	Tricuspid annulus
9	A–V node	10	S-A node
11	Tendon of Todaro	12	Bundle of His
13	Left bundle branch	14	Right bundle branch

(Triangle of Koch comprises the area between the coronary sinus, the tendon of Todaro and the tricuspid annulus)

After the impulse has been slowed in the atrio-ventricular node, propagation is rapid down the Bundle of His. These changes are reflected in the surface electrocardiogram.

Essentially the 'P' wave corresponds to atrial depolarisation, the 'P–R' interval to atrial and atrio-ventricular node conduction. The 'Q.R.S.' complex corresponds to ventricular depolarisation and the 'T' wave to ventricular repolarization. The size and shape of the various waves depend on the lead examined.

In health and at rest the heart rate is around 80 to 90 beats per minute (though in athletes it may be considerably slower), the 'P–R' interval 0.18 s, maximum 0.2 s. The 'Q.R.S' complex is of around 0.08–0.10 s duration, and the 'S.T' interval around 0.32 s. Obviously the interval between the 'T' wave of one cycle and the 'P' wave of the next is governed by the heart rate (Fig. 3.4).

Control of cardiac output

At rest the heart pumps around 5–5.5 l/min for a 70–75 kg person. This is made up of the product of a stroke volume of around 70–75 ml, pumped at a rate of 80 beats per minute. The cardiac output may also be expressed in terms of the cardiac index. This is the cardiac output per square metre of body surface area. Thus for a person of 2 square metres surface area with a cardiac output of 6 l/min the index would be 3 l/min m^2.

The pressures within the various chambers of the heart are a reflection of the volume of blood within the chamber and the tension exerted by the muscle of the wall of that chamber. The pressures within the great vessels are governed by the flow through that vessel [i.e. the cardiac output] and the resistance to flow of blood in that vessel. Some typical normal values are shown in Table 3.1.

Table 3.1   Typical pressures within a normal heart (mm Hg)

	Systolic/diastolic	Mean
Right atrium		6
Right ventricle	25/7	
Pulm. artery	25/15	15
Pulm. art. cap. wedge		10
Left atrium		10
Left ventricle	120/12	
Aorta	120/70	85

As described above, the cardiac output (Q) is a product of stroke volume and heart rate. There are several factors affecting cardiac output; venous return, mean aortic pressure, the force of contraction and the rate of contraction.

Looking first at venous return, this depends on a series of processes; Contraction of skeletal muscle and the gastro-intestinal tract forces the return of blood to the heart, both by decreasing the volume of blood held in 'capacitance' vessels and also directly increasing venous return through the muscle pump action of skeletal muscle contraction. In particular this occurs in the legs during exercise and is aided by the valves in the venous system preventing reflux of blood back into the legs. Autonomic, pharmacological and endocrine-induced venoconstriction have similar effects in increasing the tone in venous capacitance vessels and thereby increasing the venous return.

Arteriolar vasodilation and A-V shunts decrease the peripheral resistance, increasing the pressure and therefore flow in the veins, augmenting the venous return.

Mean aortic pressure can be considered as the equivalent of afterload and is a reflection of peripheral vascular resistance; if the cardiac output is kept constant, then an increase in peripheral vascular resistance will be reflected as an increase in mean aortic pressure. Conversely if the vascular resistance is decreased, then to eject a given volume of blood from the heart (stroke volume) less work will be required of the heart but the blood pressure will be lower. Following from this, if the vascular resistance is lowered and the mean aortic blood pressure kept the same, then a larger stroke volume can be ejected for the same amount of work. If the heart rate is kept fixed, then the cardiac output will be increased for the same work.

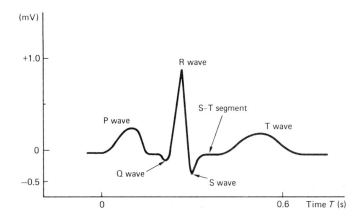

Fig. 3.4 Electrocardiogram

The force of ventricular contraction in turn depends on several factors. Firstly Starling's law shows that by increasing the end diastolic volume (EDV), and therefore the end diastolic fibre length, the stroke volume is increased. This is a reflection of a mechanical property of cardiac muscle whereby the increase in fibre length before contraction is reflected in a greater force of contraction. However, Starling's law holds only for a limited range of fibre lengths, beyond which the force of contraction declines with increasing fibre stretch. Excess ventricular filling leads to excessive ventricular dilation and a mechanical disadvantage, reflected as 'heart failure' and also to the clinically important feature of atrioventricular valve ring dilation and acute valvular incompetence. This is seen clinically for example as acute mitral incompetence in the presence of acute left heart failure.

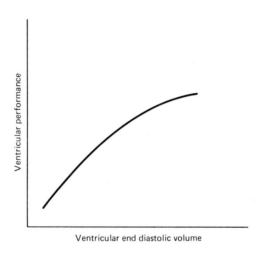

Ventricular end diastolic volume

Fig. 3.5　Ventricular performance vs EDV

In mathematical terms these changes in ventricular volume can be represented by Laplace's law, $P = 2T/R$, where P is the intraventricular pressure (end diastolic pressure) T is the wall tension and R is the radius of the ventricle (governed by the EDV). From this it can be seen that if R increases, then if T is constant P will fall, which explains part of the mechanism of ventricular dilation in heart failure. However, if P is constant, then T will increase. From these two statements we can see a further set of derivatives; if the ventricle is dilated, then the fibres will be stretched beyond the point at which Starling's law is effective and the cardiac output will fall. Mean aortic pressure will then be maintained at the expense of an increase in peripheral vascular resistance.

If the wall tension T increases, then a second complication arises: as much of coronary blood flow, particularly to the left ventricle, occurs in diastole, the rate of coronary flow depends on the gradient between aortic diastolic pressure and end diastolic intra-ventricular pressure. Increased wall tension leads to an increase in resistance to flow in coronary vessels,

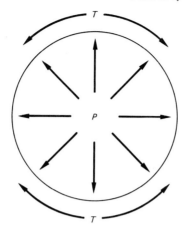

Fig. 3.6 Relation between distending pressure (P) and wall tension (T) in a hollow viscus

especially to the sub-endocardial region of the heart, and, particularly in the presence of obstructing coronary artery lesions, ischaemia and infarction can result.

Contractility or dP/dT is the change in force of contraction without change in fibre length (or EDV). It is dependent on a series of other factors: adenyl cyclase activity, increase in cAMP and increase in Ca^{2+} mobilisation and circulating hormones. Adenyl cyclase activity is stimulated by circulating adrenaline and also by increased noradrenaline production from sympathetic activity. This produces an increase in cyclic AMP production. The concentration of cAMP can also be maintained by inhibiting the enzyme responsible for its breakdown (phosphodiesterase) and drugs such as the xanthines will do this. Increase in Ca^{2+} mobilisation is dependent on increased activity in the endoplasmic reticulum. Amongst the hormones, Thyroxin, Angiotensin and Cortisol will all increase ventricular contractility.

Ventricular contractility is impaired by a further series of factors: acidosis, hypoxaemia, hyperkalaemia, hypercarbia and extremes of Ca^{2+} are the major metabolic causes. Many drugs are also potent myocardial depressants.

If the heart rate is excessively increased, then the diastolic filling time is decreased; not only is ventricular filling and hence stroke volume decrease, but coronary blood flow is impaired. All this occurs in the setting of an increase in myocardial oxygen demand. The end result is impaired ventricular contractility and the cycle of ventricular distension and further impaired contractility ensues. Table 3.2 shows factors affecting ventricular contractility.

Table 3.2 Ventricular contractility

Increased	Decreased
Sympathetic stimulation Circulating catecholamines	Parasympathetic stimulation

Hormones
  Thyroxin
  Angiotensin
  Cortisol	

Drugs
  Digoxin
  Ca++
  Beta agonists
  e.g. Adrenaline
      Isoprenaline
      Salbutamol
  Phosphodiesterase inhibitors
  e.g. Aminophylline
      Enoximone
	All other anti-arrhythmics
	
	Beta blockers

	Ischaemia Hypoxia Hyperkalaemia Hypercarbia Acidosis

4
Respiration and ventilation

The physics of respiration can be summarised in a straightforward way. Rib movement increases both the antero-posterior and lateral diameters of the thoracic cavity, whilst diaphragmatic contraction increases the cranio-caudal diameter of the thoracic cage. If the thoracic cavity were a closed system, then the increase in intrathoracic volume would be met by a decrease in intrathoracic pressure. As it is an open system, air flows into the lungs through the 'open' trachea. Expiration, during quiet breathing, is a passive process produced by elastic recoil of the lungs and chest wall. During exercise and in various pathological conditions expiration is assisted by active muscular contraction.

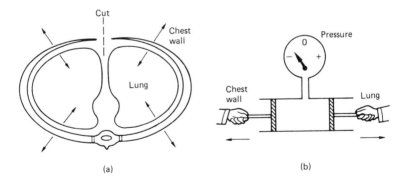

Fig. 4.1 The development of negative intrapleural pressure is due to inwards recoil force of the lungs and outwards recoil force of the chest wall. (a) The direction of these forces and the movements of the lungs and chest wall that would result if the thorax were opened. (b) A model of how intrapleural pressure is generated.

In the assessment of ventilation, there are various volumes and flows that are measured.

Firstly, the *tidal volume* (TV) is the volume of air that moves into and out of the lungs at each breath. Included in this volume is the *dead space* (DS), that part of the volume that cannot take part in respiratory gas exchange.

As can be easily appreciated, you can both inspire and expire to greater amounts than occurs in quiet respiration. Respectively the difference between the tidal volume and the volume at maximum inspiration is the *inspiratory reserve volume* (IRV), and between full expiration and the tidal volume is the *expiratory reserve volume* (ERV).

The sum of the tidal volume and the two reserve volumes, and hence the maximum volume available for use, is known as the *forced vital capacity* (FVC). It is easy to see also that at full expiration the lungs are not completely empty, the volume remaining being known as the *residual volume* (RV).

Combining the residual volume with the vital capacity produces the *total lung capacity* (TLC), which is equal to the amount of air in the lungs at full inspiration.

The *peak flow* (PF) is the fastest rate at which air can be expelled from the lungs. The *forced expiratory volume* (FEV) in the first second (FEV.1) is the total volume of air that is expelled from the lungs in the first second after initiating expiration from full inspiration. It is often expressed as a ratio to the forced vital capacity. Typical values of these various volumes are given in Table 4.1, and Fig. 4.2 shows a schematic diagram.

In restrictive lung disease, the salient feature is a reduction in total lung capacity; in obstructive lung disease the major feature is a decrease in FEV1 that exceeds the decrease in FVC. Peak flow rate is a good measure of changes in the degree of obstruction in a patient rather than being an assessment of the absolute degree of obstruction.

The rate of flow of blood through the lungs is almost equal to the cardiac output. It is important to note that there is a mismatch between the parts of the lungs that are preferentially perfused and the parts that are preferentially ventilated. This mismatch contributes to the obligatory shunt of around 5% in a normal person.

Table 4.1 Typical volumes and flows in ventilation (litres)

TV	0.4–0.6
IRV	1.9–3.3
ERV	0.7–1.0
RV	1.1–1.2
TLC	4.2–6.0
VC	3.2–4.8
DS	0.12–0.16
IC	2.4–3.8
FRC	1.8–2.2
FEV1/VC	70–80%

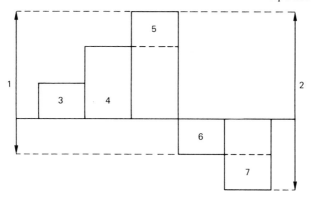

Fig. 4.2 Schematic diagram of Lung volumes

1 Vital capacity	2 Total lung capacity
3 Dead space	4 Tidal volume
5 Inspiratory reserve volume	6 Expiratory reserve volume
7 Residual volume	

At the alveolar–capillary membrane, transfer of gas from alveolus to the blood stream and vice versa is simply down the relative concentration gradients. The limiting factor is the alveolar–capillary membrane; however, as CO_2 is far more soluble than O_2 (20 times), it is normally only O_2 diffusion that is affected.

Lung compliance is a measure of the elastic recoil of the lungs and is measured as the change in unit lung volume for a fixed change in airways pressure. The normal value is around 200 ml/cm H_2O. Lung compliance is decreased in congestion, such as pulmonary oedema, ARDS and fibrotic lung disease, and increased in emphysema.

Control of respiration

The control of respiration is a complicated process, the finer points of which have yet to be fully elucidated. However, it is generally accepted that it is based around a series of feedback loops around the central automatic centre, which are both neural and chemical in nature. The central automatic centre generates both excitatory and inhibitory impulses which in turn are controlled by inhibitory feedback loops from the brain stem, regulating the pattern of respiration, and also from the cerebral cortex, which provides emotional and volitional input.

The respiratory centre itself consists of regions in the pons and medulla oblongata and contains two types of neurones. The first, the inspiratory neurones, act as a pacemaker discharge with inherent automaticity during inspiration but being inhibited by expiration. The second, the expiratory neurones, do not have spontaneous automaticity, discharge only during expiration, and are inhibited during inspiration.

Connections via the dorsal part of the central pathways project to the contralateral diaphragm through the phrenic nerve. The ventral neurones from the respiratory centre generate two sets of pathways, one to the ipsilateral phrenic nerve and the other, to both the contra and ipsilateral intercostal and accessory muscles of respiration, contains both inhibitory and excitatory fibres, thereby enabling excitation of inspiratory muscles and inhibition of the expiratory muscles, and vice versa.

Respiratory rhythm is almost certainly generated in the medulla with additional input from the pontine neurones firing in synchrony with different phases of respiration, although whether they are required for generation of rhythmic breathing remains uncertain. There is a variety of different inputs from the hypothalamus, mid-brain, vagus and other sensory sources. The overall effect of these inputs from higher centres is to smooth out the variations in respiratory pattern that would otherwise occur. Add to this inputs from cough receptors in the trachea and main bronchi, proprioceptors in muscles, tendons and joint which probably stimulate the respiratory drive at the onset of exercise and the complexity of the process becomes apparent.

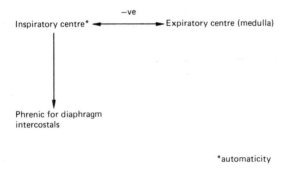

Fig. 4.3

The vagus carries a multiplicity of inputs to the respiratory centre. Stretch receptors in the lungs are activated by inflation of the lungs, impulses travelling from these receptors in the vagus to the respiratory centre are inhibitory, preventing over-inflation and limiting inflation under resting conditions. This reflex is known as the Hering–Breuer reflex.

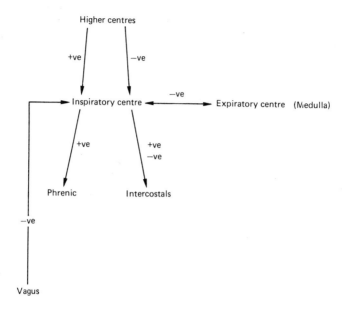

Fig. 4.4

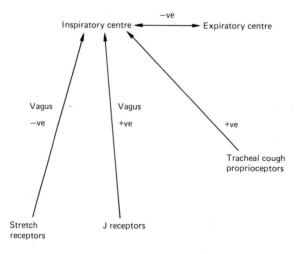

Fig. 4.5

Juxtapulmonary capillary receptors or J receptors sense pulmonary congestion. Again these send impulses back through the vagus, and their physiological role appears to be to sense increases in pulmonary capillary pressure. Unlike the stretch receptors, these stimulate respiration by their action on the respiratory centre.

The chemical control of respiration is mediated through the chemo-receptor organs located in the carotid bodies, the aorta and around the brain stem itself.

Whilst the carotid bodies sense changes in the pCO_2, pO_2 and H^+, in man the aortic bodies are sensitive only to changes in pO_2. An increase in pCO_2 or H^+ leads to an increase in ventilation, as does a fall in pO_2. The impulses are transmitted through the glossopharyngeal nerve for the carotid bodies and the vagus nerve for the aortic bodies. These impulses are excitatory to the medulla, the end effect of their actions being to hold alveolar and hence arterial pCO_2 at a constant level. Whilst the effect on the medullary chemoreceptors is similar, they are much more sensitive to changes in pCO_2 than the peripheral chemoreceptors. The effect is mediated by the sensing of changes in CSF and cerebral interstitial fluid H^+ concentrations.

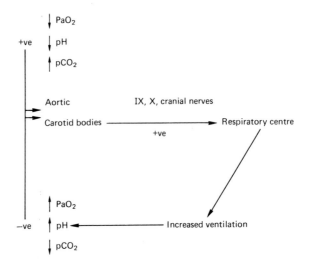

Fig. 4.6   The sensitivity of aortic and carotid chemoreceptors to a low PaO_2 is increased by the presence of a raised $PaCO_2$.

The change in the concentration of H^+ is a reflection of changes in the amount of CO_2 absorbed into solution, and hence of the pCO_2. The effect of the increase in H^+ concentration is to stimulate respiration and hence to excrete more CO_2, which results in a fall in pCO_2 and hence in CSF H^+

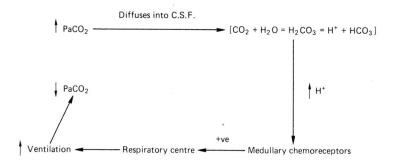

Fig. 4.7

concentration and therefore a decrease in respiratory stimulation and a return to the status quo. These effects are seen from the equation

$$CO_2 + H_2O = H_2CO_3 = H^+ + HCO_3^-.$$

5

Essential renal physiology

An understanding of renal physiology is essential on any intensive care unit and particularly on a cardiothoracic intensive care unit.

Each kidney contains over a million individual excretory units, or nephrons, which jointly receive around 20–25% of the cardiac output at rest, a figure of about 1.25 l/min, which equates to a renal plasma flow of about 0.75 l/min.

As the plasma passes through the glomerulus it is filtered to produce a filtrate. In general around 18% of the renal plasma flow is filtered to become the glomerular filtrate, producing 180 l of filtrate per 24 hours. This filtrate passes through Bowman's capsule from the glomerular capillary tuft into the tubule of the nephron. As the filtrate passes through the tubule various processes occur to modify its composition.

Firstly in the proximal tubule, water follows the osmotic gradient and moves passively out of the tubule. By the time it reaches the next part of the tubule, the Loop of Henle, around 65% of the filtered water will have been absorbed, and here a further 15% will be reabsorbed, leaving around 20% of the original water load reaching the distal tubule. In the distal tubule a further small amount of water is removed, leaving about 15% of the original glomerular filtrate to reach the collecting ducts. In the collecting duct the amount of water that is removed depends on the action of the anti-diuretic hormone ADH on the permeability of the collecting ducts to water.

Secretion of ADH increases the permeability of the collecting ducts to water, which increases the amount of water that is absorbed, which in turn decreases the amount of water that is eventually excreted. These changes in the glomerular filtrate require the maintenance of an osmotic gradient within the renal pyramids, and this results from the recirculating of solutes within the renal pyramids and the removal of water by the vasa recta, the vessels that pass through the renal pyramids.

Amongst the solute load, sodium passes from the tubular lumen into the epithelial cells, from where it is actively pumped out into the interstitial space. With it, it takes water down the osmotic gradient thus produced. There is active transport of sodium throughout the tubular system.

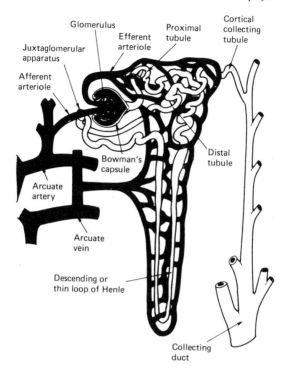

Fig. 5.1   The nephron (from Smith, The Kidney: Structure and Functions in Health and Disease. Oxford University Press, New York (1951)).

Potassium is actively absorbed in the proximal tubule, but in the distal tubule it passively moves into the tubule but is also actively secreted in exchange for sodium, which is reabsorbed. Also in the distal tubule H^+ is secreted in exchange for sodium. Hence if it is necessary to reabsorb H^+ then potassium secretion is increased. Similarly if it is necessary to retain potassium then H^+ excretion is increased.

Whilst it was thought that chloride transfer followed the movement of sodium, it is now believed that chloride is actively absorbed in the Loop of Henle.

Glucose is freely filtered in the glomerulus, at a rate dependent on its plasma concentration and up to a certain point (the tubular maximum level TMg) all is reabsorbed. This process occurs as glucose and sodium bind to a common carrier, and as sodium is reabsorbed the glucose follows into the tubular cell. It then diffuses into the interstitial fluid and then into the vasa recta.

Filtered amino acids are reabsorbed by a series of different carriers each linked to sodium reabsorption. Urea, having been filtered in the glomerulus, passes out of the tubule into the interstitium down its concentration gradient. It tends to remain in the medullary pyramids due to the vasa recta counter-current mechanisms, and hence helps to maintain the osmotic gradient of the medullary pyramid.

Creatinine is filtered in the glomerulus and in general terms the amount that is reabsorbed is balanced by the amount that is secreted into the tubular lumen.

The kidney is also an endocrine organ secreting renin, in response to hypotension and hypovolaemia. Renin release is the starting point for the renin–angiotensin–aldosterone system. Aldosterone induces sodium retention and consequently water retention, the result of this being maintenance of the circulating blood volume. The secretion of erythropoietin provides a stimulus for bone marrow production of reticulocytes and hence an adequate haemoglobin concentration.

Acid–base homeostasis

Turning now to some of the elements involved in the maintenance of pH homeostasis, there are a series of buffers in both the blood and the intracellular fluid, including haemoglobin, the carbonic acid/bicarbonate system, plasma proteins and organic phosphates.

Haemoglobin is an important buffer; firstly it is present in large quantities, secondly deoxygenated haemoglobin is a better buffer than oxygenated haemoglobin, and in addition, each molecule of haemoglobin contains 38 separate histidine groups. It is these groups that provide much of the buffering capacity in blood.

The carbonic acid/bicarbonate system is a very effective buffer system due to its ability to 'blow-off' CO_2. The buffer is described by the equilibrium; $CO_2 + H_2O = H_2CO_3 = H^+ + HCO_3^-$. The simplicity of this is that the addition of acid, i.e. H^+, to the right-hand side of the equation will produce a rebalancing of the equilibrium to the left-hand side of the equation, with an increase in CO_2 and hence pCO_2. This leads to a stimulus to respiration, and the excretion of the extra CO_2 tends to reduce the $[H^+]$ or thus bring the pH back towards normal values. Similarly an increase in CO_2 and hence pCO_2 will push the equilibrium in the opposite direction. This equation is the underlying principle for the respiratory compensation for metabolic acidosis and alkalosis. It is a 'quick response' system for changes in acid–base status, a slower compensation than occurs through the renal mechanisms. Its speed of action is dependent on the enzyme carbonic anhydrase, which catalyses the reaction

$$CO_2 + H_2O = H_2CO_3 = H^+ + HCO_3^-$$

The plasma proteins are effective buffers due to the large number of proteins and also because both their free amino and carboxyl groups

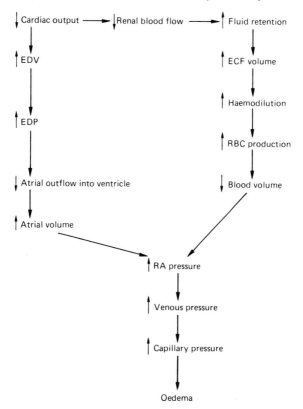

dissociate. Whilst the organic phosphates are biochemically very good buffers, due to their low concentration they contribute little to the buffering capacity in blood, although they are important buffers in the urine.

Mechanisms of oedema production

There are many causes for oedema production. These can be divided into changes in capillary permeability, changes in blood constituents and cardiac changes. Changes in capillary permeability lead to a leakage of protein into the extravascular space and loss of plasma oncotic pressure. The subsequent extravasation of water into the tissue leads to oedema. If there is a fall in plasma protein content then there is a concomitant fall in plasma oncotic pressure and movement of water from the intravascular space into the extracellular–extravascular space, and hence oedema production.

Looking in more detail at the cardiac causes of oedema, a fall in cardiac output causes a fall in renal blood flow. By the mechanisms described earlier fluid retention follows. From this ensues haemodilution, an increase in erythrocyte production, and then an increase in blood volume and right atrial pressure. From this follows an elevation in venous and capillary pressures and hence oedema as water transudes through the capillary membrane.

At the same time the fall in cardiac output leads directly to an increase in end diastolic volume and pressure, which impairs atrial outflow into the ventricle. This is followed by an increase in right atrial pressure and the same sequence of events as above.

6
The clotting mechanism

Coagulation has an interesting role in cardiac surgery: during the bypass run it is absolutely essential that complete anti-coagulation should be maintained; after the operation is completed and the coagulation corrected it becomes imperative that the patient should not bleed from non-surgical reasons. It is assumed that 'surgical' causes were excluded before the patient was closed!!

Damage to the vascular endothelium when a vessel is transected or crushed leads to the release of vasoactive substances such as prostaglandins and serotonin, which produce vaso-spasm and at the same time provide the stimulus to platelet deposition at the site of damage. Any exposed sub-endothelial tissue, in particular collagen, will also attract platelets and promote their adherence at the site of damage. The platelets undergo a release response, liberating more serotonin, ADP and other platelet factors. This produces the initial platelet plug which, even in the fully heparinised patient, will stop stitch holes bleeding.

Further reactions then are initiated in the platelet plug such that it is eventually incorporated into a clot by fibrin, the production of fibrin being a major step in haemostasis.

At the end of the coagulation cascade fibrinogen is converted into fibrin under the influence of the enzyme thrombin. Thrombin, however, is in turn created from its precursor, prothrombin, in the plasma by the action of activated factor 10 (Fig. 6.1).

However, factor 10 can be activated by two main routes. These are known as the extrinsic and intrinsic pathways. Another complication is that the enzymes named in the pathways are *not* named in numerical order. This is due to the sequence in which they were identified.

Looking at the extrinsic pathway first, inactive factor 12 is activated by exposure to collagen, which then activates factor 11 from its inactive precursor. Together with the protein Kallikrein, active factors 11 and 12 activate factor 7 from its inactive precursor. Together with calcium and tissue lipoproteins (which are released from damaged tissues and comprise tissue thromboplastin, factor 31, these activate factor 10 from its inactive precursor (Fig. 6.2).

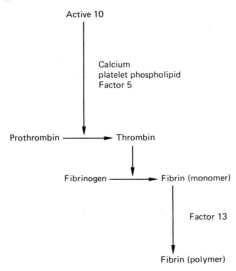

Fig. 6.1   Production of fibrin.

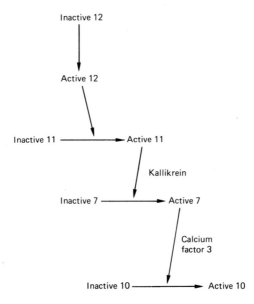

Fig. 6.2   Production of active factor 10 (extrinsic pathway).

Activated factor 10 together with platelet phospholipid, factor 5 and more calcium activates prothrombin to thrombin and the conversion of fibrinogen to fibrin monomers can then occur. However, the fibrin must then bind with other fibrin molecules to form a dense clot. This reaction requires the presence of more calcium and also factor 13.

The intrinsic pathway follows the same common path after the activation of factor 10. The differences lie in the way in which factor 10 is activated. Activation of factor 12 occurs by exposure to collagen and kallikrein, which in turn activates factor 11 from its inactive precursor. In the presence of calcium factor 11 activates factor 9. Together with more calcium, platelet phospholipid and factor 8 this complex promotes the activation of factor 10. As before, this complex with factor 5, calcium and platelet phospholipid activates prothrombin to thrombin (Fig. 6.3).

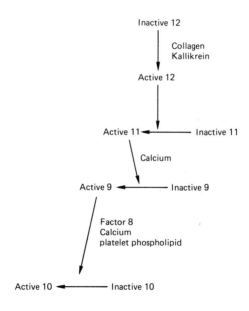

Fig. 6.3 Production of active factor 10 (intrinsic pathway).

The whole pathway can then be combined as shown in Fig 6.4.

There are a series of mechanisms that prevent unwanted intravascular coagulation and promote the dissolution of any formed intravascular clot. There is the production of anti-thrombin 3 by activated factor 10, the fibrinolytic mechanism and the inhibition of platelet aggregation by prostacyclin.

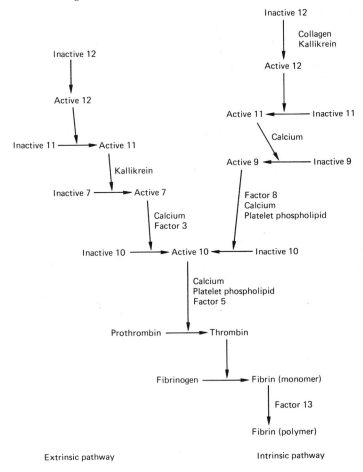

Fig. 6.4 Clotting cascade.

Anti-thrombin 3 prevents the formation of more fibrin from fibrinogen; the fibrinolytic system promotes the dissolution of clot through the production of plasmin, a fibrinolytic enzyme. Plasmin is formed from plasminogen, its precursor, by the action of a series of other agents. These include tissue plasminogen activator, thrombin and prekallikrein activators. The prekallikrein activators are formed by the action of plasmin itself on factor 12.

In clinical use the clotting cascade can be manipulated to prevent the formation of unwanted clot. Heparin acts by inhibiting the action of activated factor 9 by promoting the action of anti-thrombin 3, which inhibits the conversion of prothrombin to thrombin by activated factor 10 and the conversion of fibrinogen to fibrin under the influence of thrombin. Warfarin impedes the formation of new clotting factors (prothrombin, factors 7, 9 and 10).

Streptokinase and urokinase are plasminogen activators, as are the newer agents such as tissue plasminogen activators (rTPA) and anisoylated plasminogen streptokinase activator complex (APSAC or anistreplase).

Complement activation

Cardiopulmonary bypass has been described as a 'whole body inflammatory reaction'; this is justified by considering the mechanism and effects of complement activation during bypass.

Complement is a series of circulating glycoproteins that comprise the main pathway for action of the humoral immune response. The final effects of complement activation can be divided into three main groups; activation of coagulation and fibrinolysis, increasing vascular permeability and leucocyte phagocytosis, and target membrane lysis. There are two pathways for the activation of complement, these being described as the classical and alternative pathways. Both of these pathways possess feedback amplification loops. In the classical pathway, activation at C1 is triggered by a number of factors, the most important being antibody binding to antigen. The end result of the sequence is the production of a complex of proteins described as C56789.

In the alternative pathway, activation occurs directly at the C3 level without the previous activation of C1. There are several agents that can activate C3 at this level: these would appear to include not only endotoxins and immune complexes but also foreign materials. Evidence for this includes complement activation on bypass occurring through the alternative pathway.

Complement activation during bypass is deleterious, both directly from its 'inflammatory' effects and also by depletion of a protein that is required for normal function in the post-bypass state. Complement activation will promote histamine release, increased vascular permeability and increased leukocyte activity.

It is suggested that the leukocyte mediated pulmonary endothelial injury and the increased pulmonary capillary permeability seen after cardiopulmonary bypass may be caused by complement activation during bypass.

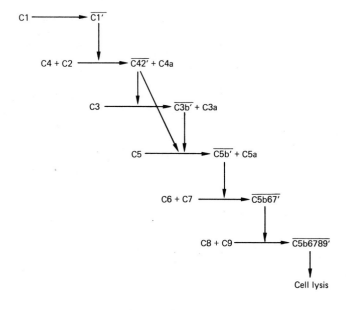

Fig. 6.5

Kinins

The kinin system is a series of basic peptides, these are activated by factor 12 which promotes the production of kallikrein from prekallikrein. In turn bradykinin is produced, which is a potent stimulus of inflammation. Kallikrein itself will also activate factor 12, as seen in the clotting cascade earlier, as well as activating plasminogen to plasmin.

7
Basic pharmacology

The receptors in the autonomic system have already been described (Chapter 2). The action of various natural and synthetic compounds at these receptors will now be described.

The sympathomimetic catecholamines produce effects that depend on their relative specificity for alpha, beta 1 and beta 2 receptors.

Adrenaline with both alpha and beta effects will produce an augmentation in heart rate, systolic blood pressure and cardiac output. In addition it produces relaxation of bronchial smooth muscle. However, these effects occur at the expense of increased myocardial oxygen demand and impaired perfusion of skin, kidneys and other viscera. It is used for its inotropic effect at doses of 1–4 μg/min (in adults), titrated according to response. In asystole it is used in intravenous boluses, usually of the 1:10 000 solution [0.1 mg/ml], and 1–5 ml will be used depending on the desperation of the situation.

Noradrenaline, with predominately alpha effects but also slight beta effects on the heart, effects an increase in both systolic and diastolic pressures, but at the cost of increased peripheral resistance and hence afterload. It increases cardiac excitability, but with little effect on cardiac output. Like adrenaline it is appropriately used in situations of hypotension associated with a low systemic vascular resistance, the classical example being septic shock. The usual intravenous rate is 1–5 μg/min (in adults) titrated against response.

Isoprenaline has predominately beta effects. Through its beta 1 effects it increases cardiac output, contractility and heart rate. There is little effect on systolic blood pressure [though it will fall acutely after an intravenous bolus, it rapidly returns to its previous level]; however, diastolic blood pressure tends to fall due to the beta 2 effects dilating the vascular beds, producing a fall in peripheral vascular resistance and afterload. The beta 2 effects also lead to a relaxation of bronchial smooth muscle. Isoprenaline is used predominately for its chronotropic effects either acutely as an intravenous bolus or as a continuous intravenous infusion. The usual bolus dose is 1–5 ml of a 1:10 000 [0.1 mg/ml] solution and as an infusion at a rate of 1–5 μg/min (in adults).

Dopamine has both alpha and beta effects together with acting on specific dopaminergic receptors. Its effects are dose dependent, though the exact dose at which different responses occur depends on the patient. At a dose of 2–5 μg/kg min it increases renal blood flow through its dopaminergic effects. At 5–10 μg/kg min its beta effects predominate with an increase in cardiac output, and above 10 μg/kg/min its alpha effects predominate with an increase in vascular resistance, including a decrease in renal blood flow and an increase in afterload.

Dobutamine is a synthetic compound, primarily a beta agonist, with more beta 1 than beta 2 activity. It also has some alpha activity. It produces relatively less tachycardia than isoprenaline or dopamine for a similar action. Dobutamine is used for its inotropic action, and is given by continuous infusion at a dose of 5–10 μg/kg/min. Its main advantage is that endogenous catecholamine stores are not depleted.

Salbutamol is a relatively specific beta 2 agonist, though it can be used for its beta 1 mediated inotropic effect. It is mostly used for its bronchodilator activity at a usual infusion rate of 5 μg/min. It is also a coronary vasodilator.

Metariminol is a relatively specific alpha agonist, usually used as an intravenous bolus in hypotension, but it can also be used by infusion. The usual bolus dose is 0.5–2.5 mg.

Phenylephrine is a relatively short acting alpha agonist which can also be useful for the management of acute hypotension, its usual dosage being 0.1–0.5 mg as an i.v. bolus.

Aminophylline, which is a phosphodiesterase inhibitor, inhibits the breakdown of cyclic AMP. As catecholamines act by the formation of cyclic AMP these two groups of compounds have potential for interaction. Aminophylline directly stimulates cardiac output but at the expense of a tachycardia. Its effect on the kidney, with an indirect increase in renal blood flow and a direct effect to decrease tubular resorption, may be of use in oliguria resistant to other agents. Aminophylline is usually used for its bronchodilator effects, the usual dose being 250 mg over 10 minutes by slow intravenous infusion, followed if necessary by an infusion at a rate of 0.5 mg/min (in adults).

Enoximone is a newer agent; it is a phosphodiesterase 4 inhibitor which exerts a positive inotropic effect, together with marked vasodilation. Its effects are not altered by alpha or beta adrenergic blockade, but they are counteracted by calcium channel blockade with verapamil. It has a long half-life and an oral preparation is available. It is possible that its effects are additive to that of beta agonists. The manufacturers recommend either initially 0.5–1.0 mg/kg by slow injection with further doses of 0.5 mg/kg at 30-minute intervals to a total initial dose of 3.0 mg/kg. Alternatively an initial infusion of 90 μg/kg/min for up to 30 minutes until the required response is achieved. Maintenance therapy is either to repeat the initial dose (up to 3.0 mg/kg) every 3–6 hours, or an infusion of 5–20 μg/kg min. Total dose in 24 hours should not usually exceed 24 mg/kg.

Alpha and beta blockers

There are two main groups of sympathomimetic receptor blocking agents of relevance. These are the alpha and beta adrenoceptor blocking agents. These drugs act by competing for receptor sites with the catecholamines. The alpha blockers tend to lower blood pressure at the expense of a compensatory tachycardia. These agents are of use in the management of post-operative hypertension, which is resistant to the more conventional agents which will be described later. Examples of alpha blockers include phenoxybenzamine, phentolamine and chlorpromazine. In the vasoconstricted patient these agents may be useful, but adequate colloid replacement should be available, as overdosage may precipitate profound hypotension.

Phentolamine is a short acting agent, usually given in a dose of 5–20 mg by intravenous injection.

Phenoxybenzamine is a longer acting agent, and a dose of 5–50 mg is usually used, given as a slow intravenous injection.

Chlorpromazine can occasionally be a useful drug in resistant hypertension. It is important to remember that its alpha blockage may become manifest if used for control of a patient with agitation after cardiopulmonary bypass.

The beta blockers are a more diverse group of drugs, which are classified into cardio- and non-cardioselective agents. In reality there is a variable degree of selectivity amongst the agents of cardio-selective groups. In pharmacological terms, they are selective for the beta 1 receptors, whereas the non-selective group act on both beta 1 and beta 2 receptors.

Examples of selective beta blockers include practolol, atenolol, acebutalol and metoprolol. The non-selective group includes oxprenolol, timolol and propranolol.

Beta blockade reduces myocardial contractility, rate of conduction of cardiac excitation and hence both cardiac output and myocardial oxygen demand. These agents tend to be used mostly for prophylaxis against, and the control of, post-operative arrhythmias. They may also be used in the control of refractory hypertension. Dosages are given in the section on class 2 anti-arrhythmic agents.

In the control of hypertension with these drugs, Labetalol has significant theoretical advantages due to its mixed alpha and beta effects. It tends to avoid the compensatory alpha-driven vasoconstriction that occurs with pure beta blockade. The usual dose is 10–50 mg by intravenous injection.

Control of hypertension in the post-operative patient is smoother with a continuous infusion technique, the commonly used agents being sodium nitroprusside and glyceryl trinitrate. Both these agents are short acting; in clinical practice the effects of glyceryl trinitrate are abolished in about two minutes and those of sodium nitroprusside in about 30 seconds. This allows rapid correction to occur in the event of an excessive hypotensive effect.

Sodium nitroprusside acts directly on the vascular smooth muscle, leading to vasodilation. Its effects are more marked in the arterial than venous vascular beds, and for this reason it tends to reduce afterload more than preload. It also has some effects as a pulmonary vasodilator. The usual infusion rate is 0.5–10 µg/kg/min.

Glyceryl trinitrate also acts directly on vascular smooth muscle; however, its effects are more pronounced as a venodilator than as an arteriodilator. For this reason it tends to reduce preload more than afterload. It also has useful effects as both a coronary and pulmonary vasodilator. The usual infusion rate is 0.5–10 µg/kg/min.

The calcium antagonist nifedipine has also been used for the control of post-operative hypertension, usually by placing the liquid from a capsule under the tongue. Control by this method appears not to be as smooth as with an intravenous infusion. It is, however, a useful agent, particularly in its slow release preparation for the control of hypertension in the late post-operative period. The usual sublingual dose is 5 mg and 10–20 mg for the slow release oral preparation.

Angiotensin-converting enzyme inhibitors

Angiotensin-converting enzyme (ACE) both converts angiotensin 1 to angiotensin 2 and also inactivates bradykinin. Angiotensin 2 has both a direct vasoconstricting effect and also produces sodium retention through the release of aldosterone. ACE inhibitors probably have their major mode of action through inhibiting peripheral conversion of angiotensin 1. Examples in clinical use at present include captopril and enalapril, both being derivatives of the amino acid proline. Both are used in hypertension and in heart failure and have similar side effects of occasional profound hypotensive episodes, impairment of renal function, neutropenia, rashes, severe angioneurotic oedema, taste disturbance and cough.

Both agents have important uses in heart failure with a decrease in left ventricular filling pressures and a reduction in both mortality and symptoms. Both may be associated with an increase in cardiac output and reduced systemic and pulmonary vascular resistances.

The usual dose is 6.25 mg p.o. increasing up to 25 mg t.d.s. for captopril and 2.5 mg p.o. increasing to 20 mg per day for enalapril. Treatment in both cases should be started in hospital.

Both these drugs are effective in hypertension, though they should not be used as the first-line treatment. Dosage is similar to that used in heart failure.

Anti-arrhythmic agents

These are best classified by their modes of action, and the Vaughan Williams classification is given below.

CLASS 1: These agents act by their membrane-stabilising effects. This includes increasing the threshold at which the cells spontaneously depolarise, decreasing the rate at which spontaneous depolarisation occurs and decreasing the rate of conduction in the conducting system.

Examples are lignocaine, tocainide, disopyramide, mexilitene, quinidine and flecainide.

CLASS 2: This group of agents act by reducing the activity of the sympathetic noradrenergic nervous system on the heart. They act by slowing the rate of spontaneous depolarisation in the pacemaker cells. The main group of compounds in this category are the beta adrenoceptor blockers.

Examples are practolol, propranolol, metaprolol and atenolol.

CLASS 3: This group consists of agents that prolong the duration of the action potential and also the effective refractory period.

Examples are amiodarone, bretyllium.

CLASS 4: This group consists of the calcium antagonists, which slow the movement of calcium ions into the cell during phase 2 of the depolarisation cycle. The effect is to reduce the excitability of pacemaker cells.

An example is verapamil.

These agents will now be looked at in more detail.

Lignocaine is a local anaesthetic agent that possesses class 1 effects as a membrane stabilising agent. Its major use is in the control of ventricular ectopic activity and in the treatment of ventricular tachyarrhythmias. It has the problems of associated hypotension, and in high doses of neurological dysfunction. This may range from confusion to fits.

It is usually used as a loading bolus of 50–100 mg, (0.75–1.5 mg/kg) followed by an infusion of 3–4 mg/min, tailing down at 1–2 hours to 1–2 mg/min depending on the control of the arrythmia.

Disopyramide, whilst having major effects as a class 1 agent, also has class 3 and 4 effects. It is useful in the control of both ventricular and supraventricular arrhythmias, though its use is complicated by its negative inotropic effect.

Intravenously, it can be used at a dose of up to 150 mg over 10–15 minutes. Like lignocaine it can also be used as an intravenous infusion at a maximum rate of 0.5 mg/min after the loading dose.

Mexilitene also has class 1 actions; like lignocaine it can be used for the management of ventricular arrhythmias. Its side effects are similar to those of lignocaine.

Intravenously it is given as a loading dose of 100–250 mg over 5–10 minutes. A further loading dose of 500 mg over the next 3–4 hours can then be followed by an infusion at a rate of 0.5 mg/min.

Flecainide has similar actions to mexilitene, but it can also have a significant negative inotropic effect.

Intravenously it is given as 2 mg/kg over 10–30 minutes to a maximum of 150 mg. This is followed by an infusion of 1.5 mg/kg/h for 1 hour decreased to 0.25 mg/kg h. The current recommendation is that it should only be used for life-threatening arrhythmias.

Amongst the Class 2 agents, the most cardioselective beta blocking agent is practolol; however, all the beta blocking agents have the side effects of hypotension and bradycardia, the non-cardioselective agents have a higher incidence of bronchospasm.

Practolol is only available for short-term intravenous use; however, in the control of supraventricular tachyarrhythmias it can be very effective.

The usual dose is 1–5 mg by slow intravenous injection, repeated as necessary.

Propranolol is a non-cardioselective agent, but it is also effective for the control of supraventricular tachyarrhythmias.

The usual dose is 1–5 mg given as a slow intranveous injection.

Other beta blockers that can be used for the control of supraventricular tachyarrhythmias include **metoprolol** and **atenolol**.

The usual dose of atenolol is 1–2.5 mg given at a rate of 1 mg/min; it can be repeated at 5–10 minute intervals to a maximum dose of 10 mg. Metoprolol is given at a rate of 1–2 mg/min to a total of 5 mg. This can be repeated to a maximum of 10 mg.

Amongst the class 3 agents, the only ones that are commonly used are amiodarone and bretyllium. Clinically these are both of use for ventricular arrhythmias, in particular sustained ventricular tachycardia, but they may also be of use in supraventricular tachycardias resistant to more conventional therapy. Side effects include hypotension and also a pro-arrhythmogenicity in certain circumstances when combined with other anti-arrhythmic agnets.

Amiodarone has several idiosyncratic side effects, ranging from unimportant corneal deposits to profound liver failure and pulmonary infiltrates. In addition it will persist in the body in tissue stores for a very long time.

The usual dose for intravenous use is a loading dose of 300 mg over 10 minutes to 3 hours, depending on the situation, followed by an infusion of 900 mg over the next 21 hours. It is usually then possible to transfer to an oral regime of 200 mg t.d.s. and measure levels after 2 or 3 days. Alternatively, further infusions of 600 mg/24 hrs can be used with monitoring of levels from the second day.

Bretyllium is given as a bolus of 100–250 mg and followed by an infusion of 0.5 mg/min.

Although there is now a wide range of class 4 agents or calcium antagonists, verapamil remains the most commonly used agent of this class for anti-arrhythmic activity.

Verapamil is of use in supraventricular tachycardias, particular atrial flutter and fast atrial fibrillation for control of ventricular rate. It has a marked negative inotropic effect and if used in the presence of previous beta blockade it may precipitate hypotension and even asystole.

The usual intravenous dose is 2.5–10 mg by very slow intravenous injection, or by infusion over 30 minutes. It can be repeated as necessary.

Cardiac glycosides

The cardiac glycosides, of which digoxin is the best known, but also include digitoxin, digitalis and ouabaine, are used in the management of supraventricular arrhythmias, in particular atrial fibrillation. The effects are initiated through depression of the rate of conduction in the conducting system, and by increased vagal activity.

In atrial fibrillation these effects are mostly due to delay in conduction through the atrioventricular node; however, conversion of atrial flutter to fibrillation may occur due to an increase in the atrial refractory period. The action of digoxin is mediated through its inhibition of a sodium–potassium ATPase enzyme, leading to an increase in intracellular calcium. Hypokalaemia potentiates the effect of digoxin and may precipitate toxicity.

The usual loading dose of digoxin is 0.75 mg/M^2 body surface area. This is generally given in divided doses over 8–15 hours, but it can be given much more quickly if needed.

It is important to remember that digoxin toxicity can manifest as either atrial or ventricular arrhythmias, and therefore digoxin levels should be checked after treatment has been started. These should lie between 1.5 and 2.5 µg/l. It is now possible to treat severe digoxin toxicity with specific monoclonal antibodies.

Analgesia and anti-emetics

The most commonly used agent for post-operative pain control is papaveretum ('Omnopon'). Other members of the opioid group are used as is the synthetic agent buprenorphine. From 48 hours after surgery most patients can be controlled with an oral agent, such as the compound preparations of paracetamol and dihydrocodeine or dextropropoxyphene.

Papaveretum is a mixture of opium alkaloids, with pharmacology similar to that of morphine. On the brain it induces a state of relaxation and euphoria, together with sleepiness. Importantly this group of drugs depress respiration by reducing sensitivity to an increase in pCO_2. On the cardiovascular system the major side effects that are occasionally seen are hypotension and bradycardia which usually respond to volume replacement. Commonly they also produce delayed gastric emptying in association with nausea and constipation from direct effects on smooth muscle in the gut. The effects of overdosage can be reversed with the antagonist naloxone.

Papaveretum is usually used in 1–5 mg intravenous boluses, as an intravenous infusion of 1–5 mg/h, or as 10–20 mg intramuscular injections.

Naloxone is used in 0.2 mg intravenous increments, repeated as necessary.

For post-operative antiemetics, the usual drugs of choice are metoclopramide or prochlorperazine.

Metoclopramide acts by inhibiting the chemoreceptor trigger zone for vomiting and also through direct effects relaxing the pyloric sphincter and increasing gastric emptying.

It is usually given at a dose of 5–10 mg intravenously or intramuscularly every 4 hours as necessary.

Prochlorperazine is a phenothiazine derivative that acts through central mechanisms to inhibit vomiting.

It is given as a dose of 12.5 mg 4–6 hourly.

Paralysis is sometimes necessary and the non-depolarising agent pancuronium is a useful first line agent.

Pancuronium is given as an initial dose of 6–8 mg followed by 2–4 mg increments as required.

For sedation as opposed to analgesia the benzodiazepine group of drugs are useful. The commonest agents used are diazepam and midazolam.

Midazolam is given as a dose of 1–5 mg by intravenous bolus injection. This can be repeated or alternatively an infusion of 3–5 mg/h can be started.

Diazepam is given as a dose of 5–20 mg repeated as necessary.

Both these agents may cause hypotension which usually responds to volume replacement.

Flumazenil is a new agent that acts as a specific benzodiazepine antagonist. Initial dose is 200 μg, with further 100 μg boluses given up to a total of 2 mg in an intensive care. It can be given as an intravenous infusion of 100–400 μg/h.

Propofol is a new anaesthetic induction agent that is used in some units for up to 24 hours of sedation when given by intravenous infusion.

Diuretics

Diuretics are part of the basic therapy of cardiac disease, and the most commonly used on the ICU are the loop diuretics. These act by inhibiting sodium reabsorption in the Loop of Henle. However, as they present a greater sodium load in the distal Loop of Henle they lead to impaired potassium retention and a net potassium loss. Examples of this group include the following.

Frusemide is used at a starting dose of 10 to 20 mg iv and increased as necessary.

Bumetanide is used at a dose of 0.25 to 2 mg iv and increased as necessary.

Ethacrynic acid is used at a dose of 25 to 50 mg by slow intravenous infusion.

In resistant oliguria, the osmotic diuretic mannitol is useful, especially if the blood volume is not thought to be overloaded.

Mannitol is used at a dose of 10–20 g (50–100 ml of 20% solution) repeated as necessary.

As previously discussed, dopamine at a dose of 2–5 μg/kg/min is an effective diuretic agent.

Aminophylline at a dose of 125–250 mg by slow intravenous injection can also be used.

Metalozone is derived from the thiazide group of agents; it is very active when used orally, in general at a dose of 5 mg, 2 or 3 times a week.

Antibiotics

Antibiotic prophylaxis is an essential part of modern cardiac surgery. Most units give the first dose at induction, and then carry on for a variable time, usually 2–5 days.

For the routine coronary artery bypass graft, the regime usually consists of 48 hours of intravenous therapy alone. In many units the same regime is used for valve surgery as well; in others a further 3–5 days of the equivalent oral antibiotics are continued.

The exact details of prophylaxis vary from unit to unit, depending on local sensitivities. The aim is to prevent infection of sternal and leg wounds and, most importantly, of implanted prosthetic valves and other material. Staphylocci are the most feared contaminants in cardiac surgery; prosthetic valve endocarditis has a very high mortality. A common regime is **flucloxacillin** 500 mg 6 hourly, with either **gentamicin** 1 mg/kg 8–12 hourly and **benzylpenicillin** 600 mg 6 hourly or **cephradine** 500 mg 6 hourly. Either regime should give good cover but should be reviewed in the light of local knowledge.

The major side effects of the penicillins are anaphylaxis, whereas gentamicin is both oto- and nephrotoxic. Gentamicin levels should be checked in patients with renal impairment, and in those whose therapy exceeds 48 hours.

In the case of known penicillin sensitivity, then **erythromycin** 500 mg 6 hourly is an alternative.

Drugs and clotting

Heparin is an organic acid mucopolysaccharide, occurring naturally in mast cells. In vivo, high concentrations are found in the liver and also in the lung. It is a supremely effective anti-coagulant, which works by promoting the action of anti-thrombin 3. Anti-thrombin 3 inhibits the action of activated factor 10 (factor 10a) as well as inhibiting the conversion of fibrinogen to fibrin under the influence of thrombin.

The major complication of its use is bleeding from excessive and uncontrolled dosage. It is given as a continuous intra-venous infusion when used over a long time, but as a single bolus when given before the institution of cardiopulmonary bypass.

Its dosage can be controlled by a number of different tests, in particular the thrombin time, the activated partial thromboplastin time and the activated clotting time. For both the thrombin time and the partial thromboplastin time, full anti-coagulation is achieved when the times are prolonged to three times normal. The activated clotting time is used for the control of heparinisation on bypass, and should be greater than 450 before bypass is instituted. It should have returned to the pre-operative control value, usually around 125, after the effects of heparin have been reversed with protamine.

The usual dosage at the onset of bypass is around 300 units per kilogram (1 mg/kg).

Protamine is a strongly basic protein, which combines with heparin to form a stable but inactive complex.

Its usual dose after bypass is 10 mg per thousand units of heparin given and then the activated clotting time is checked and more given as necessary. An alternative strategy is to give 1 mg protamine for each milligram of heparin that was given.

Side effects include rashes, hypotension, bradycardia and acute pulmonary hypertension.

Warfarin is an anti-coagulant of the coumarin class, and acts by impeding the formation of factors 2, 7, 9, 10 from vitamin K by the liver. Whilst heparin was discovered by an astute medical student (Maclean in 1916) the coumarins were discovered after mouldy clover was identified as the cause of a curious bleeding diathesis in cattle. Due to the action of warfarin in impeding the formation of new clotting factors it has a much slower onset of action as well as taking much longer for its action to wear off. Its effect can be measured through the prothrombin time. Usually this will be kept at between 2.5 and 3 times its control value.

Its usual dosage for long-term use will be between 3 and 6 mg but can vary widely depending on liver function.

The effects of warfarin can be reversed with fresh frozen plasma, which contains factors 1 (fibrinogen), 2 (prothrombin), 7, 9, 10. Alternatively if reversal is not urgent then vitamin K can be given. However, if further warfarinisation is to be required it may prove difficult to control initially.

Like heparin, excessive bleeding is the most common problem, though allergic reactions, usually rashes, do occur.

Streptokinase, like urokinase, is a plasminogen activator. Its action therefore is to promote fibrinolysis and hence if used after a surgical procedure it may cause bleeding from previously haemostatic suture lines. It is used in the treatment of established thrombosis, such as a coronary artery thrombosis or a pulmonary embolus. It is not used in the prophylaxis of thrombosis, nor in the establishment of routine anti-coagulation.

Anisolyated plasminogen streptokinase activator complex (APSAC/ anistreplase) is a modification of streptokinase. Not only is it a pro-drug that is progressively de-acylated with a half-life of around 90 minutes and hence has a prolonged period of action, but also as it provides a preformed plasminogen–streptokinase complex, it enhances the formation of plasmin at its target sites. It is being used for the acute therapy of myocardial infarction.

Recombinant **tissue plasminogen activator** has recently been released. It is a glycoprotein that activates the conversion of plasminogen to plasmin.

It is being used for the acute therapy of myocardial infarction. Its use before surgery may lead to prolonged bleeding.

Vitamin K, which occurs in two forms in nature (K1 and K2) is a fat soluble vitamin, absorbed only in the presence of bile salts. It is essential for the production of factors 2, 7, 9 and 10, its deficiency in liver disease will manifest firstly as a haematological and subsequently as a clinical impairment of clotting.

Anti-fibrinolytic agents

Tranexamic acid and **epsilon amino caproic acid** are the clinically used examples of this class of agents. They act by inhibiting the action of plasmin to breakdown fibrin, (fibrinolysis). In clinical practice they are sometimes of use in the slow ooze that may be seen after surgery.

Anti-platelet agents

Aspirin is an anti-platelet agent, which acts by inhibiting the production of thromboxane A2 during platelet formation. As a result, there is impairment of both platelet adherence and aggregation, consequently global platelet function is impaired. In addition to this platelet function is impaired by the cardiopulmonary bypass run and it would appear that patients who have had aspirin in the immediate pre-operative period tend to bleed more heavily after their operation.

Dipyridamole has an anti-platelet activity which is manifest through its inhibition of phosphodiesterase and also through a stimulation of platelet adenyl cyclase formation. It is usually used with aspirin in an attempt to reduce the incidence of late vein graft occlusion. It may be poorly tolerated due to nausea as well as causing headaches through its vasodilator effects.

Prostacyclin acts by increasing platelet cyclic AMP and hence inhibiting platelet aggregation. It also dilates vascular smooth muscle, in particular it will lower both pulmonary and systemic vascular resistance. Side effects include nausea, asthma and excessive bleeding.

Aprotinin is a protease inhibitor that has recently been shown in high doses to be effective in preventing platelet activation during cardiopulmonary bypass. After the reversal of heparin with protamine, platelet function appears to be near normal and blood loss is significantly reduced. It is suggested that the mode of action is to prevent platelet activation in the bypass tubing and oxygenator. It is currently available only on a named patient basis for this indication. However, it is an inhibitor of the fibrinolytic activity of the plasmin-streptokinase complex, formed after thrombolytic therapy with streptokinase, and is available generally for this use.

8
Nutrition

Feeding and nutrition is never an emergency, therefore there will always be time for reflection and discussion on the best routes and forms of nutrition for the post-surgical patient. In general the routine patient will be extubated on the night of the operation, take sips of water on the first post-operative morning and manage a light breakfast on the second day, by which time all his or her intravenous lines will have been removed. For these patients the provision of nutrition is not a problem.

The energy requirements of the septic, catabolic patient are very different. However, even in the worse case the energy requirements will not exceed twice the basal metabolic requirement for any particular patient. An adult in bed at rest needs 25 kcal/kg body mass (1875 kcal for a 75 kg man) and therefore will need at most 50 kcal/kg when severely catabolic (3750 kcal for a 75 kg man). Most patients with problems on the ICU will need between 30 and 40 kcal/kg/day. Glucose provides 4 kcal/g. Optimum utilisation occurs when it is administered at a rate of 5 mg/kg/min (540 g/day for a 75 kg man), in practice it is not usually used at a rate exceeding 3 mg/kg/min.

Baseline nitrogen requirement is 250 mg nitrogen per kilogram body mass per day. As 1 g nitrogen corresponds to 6.25 g protein this corresponds to 1.5625 g protein/kg (18.75 g nitrogen and 117 g protein per day for a 75 kg man). However, under stress the nitrogen requirements will increase up to 400 mg/kg/day, which corresponds to 2.5 g protein/kg/day (this is 30 g nitrogen per day or 187.5 g protein per day for a 75 kg man).

In practice it is rare to use more than 20 g nitrogen per day. The standard synthetic solutions provide 4 kcal/g.

There are essential requirements for fatty acids and these are usually supplied as lipid emulsions. These will provide 9 kcal/g.

The precise requirements of vitamins and minerals are difficult to define, but include not only replacement of water and fat-soluble vitamins but also minerals including zinc, phosphate and magnesium.

The maximum energy that can be provided by glucose is limited as high infusion rates cause a rise in noradrenaline secretion, an increase in O_2

consumption and an increase in CO_2 production. In practice the maximum energy that can be safely and effectively delivered by a glucose infusion is 2000 kcal per day. Much of the rest of the energy requirement can be delivered in a fat emulsion and the remainder as part of amino acids or protein.

Insulin is important in nutrition as it not only maintains normoglycaemia but also promotes protein anabolism. In particular the uptake of amino acids and protein synthesis by muscle is facilitated.

The easiest assessment of nutritional status is to measure the serum albumin concentration. A level below 21 g/l represents severe malnutrition, between 21 and 28 g/l is moderate and above 28 g/l and below 35 g/l is mild malnutrition.

The way in which nutrition can be delivered to patients depends on their gastro-intestinal function. Those patients with GI motility and absorption can be fed through the enteral route, either orally, through a naso-gastric tube or even a feeding jejunostomy. However, in the absence of GI function then the parenteral route must be used.

There is a wide range of proprietary solutions available for feeding through both the enteral and parenteral routes. For each route these solutions can be manipulated to provide the optimum treatment for each patient. The fluid volume and electrolyte requirements of the patient must be assessed on at least a daily basis and adjusted according to the clinical, biochemical and haemodynamic parameters. Vitamin, mineral, trace elements and folate replacement therapy should be used routinely in patients undergoing long-term feeding, particularly in those undergoing parenteral nutrition.

The effectiveness of therapy in the clinical setting is best monitored by daily weight, the absence of tissue oedema, the level of plasma albumin and transferrin. There are many other more complex methods but for the moment they remain research tools.

Enteral nutrition is best provided through a fine bore naso-gastric feeding tube and a constant infusion rate pump. Parenteral nutrition should be provided through a separate, dedicated, tunnelled silastic feeding line. The usual site of insertion is into the superior vena cava through a sub-clavian approach. It must be inserted and handled with meticulous attention to asepsis.

In practice in many units the management of parenteral nutrition is becoming the preserve of a separate subspecialty, that will assess and manage these problems.

9

Pre-operative assessment

The importance of the pre-operative assessment cannot be overstated; errors of diagnosis and of management will lead to an immense degree of stress to all involved. Major ICU morbidity can often be predicted from pre-operative risk factors.

Assessment starts with a carefully taken history, with emphasis not only on the presenting condition but also on operative risk factors. As an example, coronary artery disease is almost invariably associated with smoking and hence with chronic obstructive airways disease, therefore a careful assessment of sputum production is useful. A previous history of cerebral vascular disease would suggest the need not only for even more careful palpation of the aorta at cannulation but also consideration of running at a higher flow during the cardiopulmonary bypass run than might otherwise be chosen.

Obviously a history of varicose veins or their surgery has great implications for vein harvesting in coronary artery surgery, but even in non-coronary surgery it is important to know; just occasionally some vein will be needed both unexpectedly and in a hurry. A history of unilateral claudication would suggest the use of the opposite leg for vein harvesting and thus leaving the long saphenous in place for future peripheral vascular surgery.

In the cardiac history itself one should always be on the lookout for atypical features; multiple episodes of pain in coronary artery disease is occasionally due to pericarditis, which can cause an unpleasant surprise on opening the chest. Shortness of breath is occasionally due to a carcinoma of the lung rather than increasing heart failure.

Examination of the patient will invariably concentrate on the cardio-vascular and respiratory systems, but again unexpected surprises may turn up anywhere. Features of importance include the pulse, particularly the carotid, its rate rhythm and character and the blood pressure. The apex beat should be palpated and then the heart can be auscultated.

The respiratory system should be examined, not only as a diagnostic procedure but also as a baseline for comparison with its post-operative condition.

Examine the abdomen with care as the incidence of abdominal aortic aneurysms and carcinomas of the colon in this age group is appreciable. The nervous system should not be ignored and as a final move, stand the patient up, examine the legs and the long saphenous veins.

The ECG, both resting and exercise, and CXR must be reviewed, then the routine haematology and electrolytes. The echo-cardiogram should be examined not only looking at the ventricular function, but also for unexpected valve calcification and if doppler echo is available for valve gradients. Other non-invasive studies such as radio-isotope regional perfusion and ventriculography studies should be checked and finally the cardiac catheter and angiogram reviewed.

The cardiac catheter and angiogram allow an accurate estimation of intra-cardiac pressures, of ventricular function, and coronary anatomy. In paediatric heart disease it is an adjunct to echo-cardiography in demonstrating the cardiac morphology and intracardiac connections. Apart from the diagnostic function, it is also becoming a therapeutic tool with a range of techniques from atrial septostomy and pulmonary valvotomy in neonates to mitral valvuloplasty in the elderly.

Cardiac catheterisation may simply be confined to the left side of the heart or may include right-sided studies as well. The decision as to which sides are studied depends on the expected diagnosis based on the pre-catheter work-up. A patient with uncomplicated angina and a positive exercise test will simply undergo a left heart study with measurement of left ventricular end diastolic pressures, left ventricular and aortic pressures. (LVEDP, LV, Ao.) A right heart study will be indicated in patients with right-sided lesions, shunts, and in whom pulmonary hypertension or raised pulmonary vascular resistance might be expected.

The LVEDP is an index of ventricular performance; in the absence of mitral stenosis it correlates with left atrial pressures, and its elevation suggests an impairment of left ventricular performance.

Pulmonary hypertension and a raised PVR imply either a primary pulmonary hypertension or more commonly a secondary effect to either raised left atrial pressure, increased pulmonary blood flow or alveolar hypoxia.

Cardiac angiography is used to demonstrate the intra-cardiac anatomy, most commonly at present to demonstrate coronary anatomy and the site of stenotic lesions. This allows a decision to be made on the indications for surgery, which vessels are to be grafted and the site at which those grafts will be inserted.

10
The transfer to the ICU

The transfer to the intensive care unit from the operating theatre is the most unstable time in the patient's post-operative course. Having been cold and vasoconstricted on the operating table during the bypass run, the patient has started to warm up towards the end of the procedure and this continues during the transfer. At the time of the transfer the monitoring is often less comprehensive than it has been in theatre – the minimum must be a continual ECG trace and an arterial waveform and pressure display.

From the anaesthetic point of view many of the patients being transferred will be intubated and ventilated, and therefore the airway must be maintained and the patient adequately ventilated at all times. It is traditional that the drains are clamped during transfer to prevent the development of a pneumothorax should they accidently become disconnected. This is not necessary: even if the pleura has been breached, expansion of the lungs is maintained by the compression of the bag by the anesthetist. In addition, if the patient should suddenly bleed during the transfer not only will this not be immediately appreciated by the sudden increase in blood loss but also the patient may rapidly arrest from the effects of cardiac tamponade.

When the patient is received onto the ICU by the resident, details of the procedure that has been undertaken should be checked, together with any untoward events. In particular the nature of any inotropic support and the reasons for its use should be discussed. It is worth knowing if there has been excessive bleeding since cardiopulmonary bypass was discontinued, as transfusion since then may not have been adequate. It is worth checking at this time the sites to which drains and any pacing wires have been placed.

The plan for ventilation should be discussed at this time and the aim is usually for rapid extubation. Obviously, this is not so if the patient is bleeding excessively, has very poor blood gases or is otherwise unstable. In an ICU the time of the night alone should not be an indication to sedate a patient for extubation at a more convenient hour.

The pulse, blood pressure, and ventilator settings will be checked by the nurse looking after the patient as the patient is received onto the ICU and the resident should ensure that the patient's condition is satisfactory. By this time the patient will have been connected to the monitoring systems and this will include continuous ECG, arterial, central venous and occasionally direct or indirect left atrial pressure monitoring.

Apart from the dynamic real time monitoring, the patient's observations will be recorded at regular intervals. This will be at every 15 minutes for the first couple of hours or until the patient is stable and then every 30 minutes for a further couple of hours or until the patient is stable. If the signs are stable at this time then the recordings will become hourly.

The importance of these records is that they allow the identification of developing trends and the early management of problems. In time these observations will be superseded by the new forms of computerised monitoring and data management that are being developed.

The monitoring of urine output is one of the mainstays in the assessment of the cardiac output; however, as cardiac surgery has become more commonplace and patients are extubated earlier, the catheterisation of patients has, in some centres, stopped being routine. Obviously, in patients in whom a difficult or prolonged procedure is anticipated, catheterisation should be performed pre-operatively. Non-catheterised patients who return to the ICU on inotropes and those in whom ventilation is prolonged should be catheterised on the ICU.

Once the patient is on the ICU, then the various management orders can be assessed. It is helpful to think of these under different headings:

(1) **Colloid**. There are various ways of writing these orders. It is simplest to think of the task in two components; firstly replace losses from the chest drains, and then give colloid to fill up the intravascular space as the patient warms up and consequently dilates. This gives a measure of the amount of colloid that has been given in excess of blood losses, or 'blood balance', and depending on the temperature at which the patient arrived on the ICU this is not normally much above 750 ml. The order then will usually be written as

1. Own blood, 2. Plasma expander (maximum 1000 ml), 3 Donor blood. To keep CVP at . . . to . . . mm Hg.

In this way the least amount of bank blood is used.

(The figures selected will depend on the cardiac performance in theatre. Alternatively PACWP or Left Atrial pressures can be used.)

(2) **Crystalloid**. This will be given as either 5% dextrose or dextrose–saline and, depending on the type of prime used for the bypass circuit, this will usually be infused at a rate of 0.5–0.75 ml/kg/h. It will include all the fluid used as transport for the various drugs that are given. The order then can be written as

Crystalloid, 5% dextrose to total of . . . ml/h.

(3) **Hypotensives and vasodilators**. These have two main functions, firstly by reducing both preload and afterload they will reduce myocardial work and hence myocardial oxygen demand, and secondly by promoting vasodilation they allow the patient to be transfused up to an appropriate circulating volume more rapidly.

The two more commonly used agents are sodium nitroprusside and glyceryl trinitrate. Of the two SNP is the more effective for the control of hypertension, and GTN the more effective for reducing preload. GTN has the additional useful advantage of being a coronary vasodilator. The orders can be written as

GTN 50 mg in 100 ml at 0–20 ml/h to keep systolic blood pressure below 110 mm Hg. If necessary add SNP 50 mg in 100 ml at 0–20 ml/h.

(4) **Inotropes**. The choice of inotrope depends on the situation, and frequently on local preference. Their use will depend on the requirements of each patient; taking dopamine as an example, it can be given to maintain an adequate blood pressure. The concentration at which it is made up will depend on local practice – the example here is given for a 75 kg patient:

Dopamine, 200 mg in 100 ml 5% dextrose, give at 4–7 μg/kg/min (9–16 ml/h) to keep systolic blood pressure at 100–110 mm Hg.

It is often safer if once an infusion rate has been established for it to be weaned gradually once the patient has stabilised rather than arbitrarily turning down the infusion, and this can be written as

Dopamine, wean by 1 μg/kg/h every hour providing systolic blood pressure remains over 100 mm Hg.

If this combination is unsuccessful then the ICU resident should be informed as further assessment will be necessary.

(5) **Analgesia**. There are essentially two options, either a continuous infusion technique or intermittent small intravenous boluses. Providing the intermittent boluses are given frequently enough or the infusion is given at an adequate rate there should be little to choose between the two methods. However, in practice, the continuous infusion technique is generally more convenient and provides a better level of analgesia. The orders can be written as

Papaveretum, 60 mg in 60 ml at 0–6 ml/hr, by continuous infusion, or
Papaveretum, 2.5–5 mg by intermittent intravenous bolus.

(6) **Anti-emetics**. If a Ryles tube has been passed, which is not routine, then aspiration is often the quickest method of relief. However, an anti-emetic should always be prescribed; Metoclopramide 10 mg 4 hourly by i.v. bolus is a useful agent.

Histamine H2 receptor antagonists are prescribed if there is evidence of previous symptoms of gastric ulceration or dyspepsia.

(7) **Potassium replacement**. This is used for its anti-arrhythmic activity, the optimum serum potassium being between 4.5 and 5.0 mmol/l. Its order can be written as

KCl, 10–20 mmol in 20 ml over 20 minutes by intravenous infusion, to keep serum potassium between 4.5 and 5.0 mmol/l.

Monitoring on the ICU

Monitoring on the ICU takes many forms; at its most simple it consists solely of serial pulse recordings; at its most invasive it will include arterial, right and left atrial pressure and thermodilution cardiac output monitoring.

For post-operative cardiac surgery, the minimum necessary monitoring is axillary temperature, ECG with numerical heart-rate display, right atrial and arterial pressure waveforms together with an accurate numerical display. The monitoring of urine output is discussed below.

These are all dynamic real-time measurements which are then recorded usually onto paper charts, though the era of computerised monitoring and storage is rapidly dawning. Apart from displaying the current state of a patient the recordings allow an assessment of trends in a patient's status and early action to improve a deteriorating state.

Pulse rate and rhythm are easily seen on a simple ECG monitor; this allows immediate visualisation of rhythm abnormalities though a full 12 lead recording may be necessary for the assessment of complex rhythm disturbances. Together with measurement of respiratory rate and temperature these are the simplest level of monitoring.

In the extubated patient respiratory rate and the pattern of ventilation will vary under differing physiological stresses; whilst the patient in pain will take rapid and shallow breaths, the over-narcotised patient will take slow, shallow and often irregular breaths.

Catheterisation and regular monitoring of urine output is essential in the patient who is receiving inotropic therapy or who has an element of renal impairment or is on long-term (more than 6 hours at the most) ventilation. Changes in the urine output over several hours are often a reflection of the varying cardiac output. In the routine CABG patient it is debatable whether the risks of both sepsis and urethral strictures do not outway the benefits of measuring urine output.

Temperature changes are very important in the patient who has just undergone a cardiopulmonary bypass. All such patients will return to the ICU with some degree of hypothermia and as they wake up and are transfused with colloid their temperature should return to normal or mildly elevated levels. Failure to do this, with a low central venous pressure, in the face of apparently adequate volume replacement is highly suggestive of occult bleeding and suggests the need for a chest x-ray. A low temperature with adequate volume replacement, a rising central venous pressure and a low blood pressure is highly suggestive of a low cardiac output state. This may be due simply to a need for inotropic support or it may reflect a state of cardiac tamponade.

Central venous pressure monitoring is used for an assessment of the amount of colloid required to replace losses, both as the patient bleeds and also as the patient warms up. In general, adequate circulation should be achieved with a CVP of 5–15 mm Hg. If the patient remains hypotensive at this level, then judicious further transfusion should be attempted and a failure of response suggests the need for inotropic support. A grossly elevated CVP suggests the presence of tamponade and the need for further assessment. A fall in blood pressure in the face of a 200 ml colloid challenge is highly suggestive of tamponade. Falsely elevated CVP readings may occur from an obstructed or kinked cannula and this should always be checked. Often the easiest way of doing this is to display the pressure trace on a monitor.

Continuous arterial pressure monitoring not only allows second by second monitoring of blood pressure but also gives easy access for serial blood gas analysis. Continuous blood pressure monitoring is essential during the bypass run and the facility is easily transferred back to the ICU. Its use allows the accurate titration of colloid replacement, hypotensive and inotropic agents. The facility for easy arterial blood sampling and the estimation of pO_2, pCO_2 and acid-base status is essential in the careful and accurate management of these patients.

In the sicker patient more invasive monitoring becomes necessary. This is usually an attempt to measure left atrial filling, left ventricular function and cardiac output. At operation it is easy to insert a left atrial pressure line into the left atrium, either through the right superior pulmonary vein or through the right atrial purse string and across the atrial septum. It is possible to pass a pulmonary artery line through the right atrium and ventricle and into the pulmonary artery.

The left atrial line allows a direct measurement of left ventricular filling and left ventricular end diastolic pressure, from which manipulations can be made to reduce diastolic wall tension and optimise coronary artery perfusion. The aim of this is to avoid sub-endocardial ischaemia.

The pulmonary artery pressure line is an alternative to a pulmonary artery flotation catheter in adults; however, it is usually used in neonatal and paediatric surgery.

The thermodilution pulmonary artery catheter in adults provides facilities for measuring left atrial pressure through the pulmonary artery capillary wedge pressure. It allows a direct measurement of pulmonary artery pressures and through the thermodilution technique it allows estimation of cardiac output. It is inserted as a percutaneous procedure through cannulation of a large vein, generally the internal jugular though the subclavian is an alternative. The pulmonary artery diastolic pressure is usually 2–4 mm Hg higher than the pulmonary artery capillary wedge pressure.

Assessment of cardiac output

Cardiac output may be assessed both by indirect clinical parameters and by direct measurement. The clinical features of the low output state include cool peripheries with low volume pulses and slow venous return in a sweaty patient. Agitation and confusion may also be present. In children circumoral pallor and puckering may also be present.

Measurements of urine output will show a fall in urine output to less than 0.5 ml/kg/min; the blood pressure will generally be low, often less than 100 mm Hg systolic. The CVP should be low if the aetiology is simply hypovolaemia, but elevated in cardiac failure or tamponade.

The mixed venous oxygen tension and saturation will be reduced ($PMV.O_2 < 4$ kPa (30 mm Hg) and saturation $< 60\%$), as may be the arterial pO_2. The fall in $PMV.O_2$ is a reflection of increased tissue oxygen extraction in the presence of local tissue acidosis.

Arterial blood gas analysis will show an acidosis, often with a pH of < 7.2 and a base excess of > -5 mmol/l. Plasma bicarbonate will be reduced to < 20 mmol/l.

The cardiac output can be measured directly by various techniques including Doppler ultrasound techniques and pulmonary artery thermo-dilution catheters.

The critical level for survival requires the cardiac index (cardiac output divided by body surface area) to be maintained at over 2.2 l/min/M2. If it falls below this for more than 24 hours then the mortality approaches 100%.

Post-operative chest X-ray

In the post-operative chest X-rays there are several important initial observations to be made. Firstly although there will usually be previous films for comparison, the ITU films are usually taken in the antero-posterior view and at a variable distance from the patient, so assessment of change in the width of the mediastinum and hence the presence of blood clot after surgery can be difficult. Secondly many of these films are taken in the supine position and so will not show the classical meniscus of fluid in the costo-phrenic angles; however, the presence of fluid will be suspected by a general 'haziness' which will be more obvious if it is unilateral.

A scheme that includes the following points should be followed: check the name and date of the X-ray together with the side marker. Next check the penetration of the film and for the presence of rotation. Now is a good time to check the position of any vascular catheters and intra-pleural drains. Check that the endotracheal tube if present is placed such that its end lies above the carina and then look at the position of the media-stinum; in particular check that it is not deviated to either side. Usually the position of the trachea itself is the best guide to deviation of the mediastinum.

Next look at the position of the two hilar shadows; if one or other of these are swung down it suggests the presence of at least some lower lobe collapse. Next look at the costophrenic angles, as the presence of fluid will cause 'blunting' of these angles in the film taken in the erect position. Now exclude a pneumothorax by checking the lung markings.

Looking at the lung fields, a generalised haziness could be due to pulmonary oedema or fluid in both hemi-thoraces, whilst unilateral haziness is more likely to signify fluid, often blood, in the hemi-thorax. If upper lobe blood diversion is present, then it is significant of left ventricular failure.

Sequential enlargement of the cardiac shadow over a series of films indicates the need for an echo-cardiogram to exclude an intrapericardial collection of blood or fluid.

11
Techniques

All of the procedures to be detailed here are invasive and should be treated as sterile procedures; at the very least gloves should be worn. For the more major procedures a mask and gown are required.

(1) Subclavian approach for insertion of central lines

Explain to the patient what you are about to do.

Place the patient in a flat or mild head-down position, and clean with iodine or similar an area extending from the opposite sternoclavicular joint to the acromioclavicular joint on the side on which you are working. This area should be extended up to the angle of the jaw and down to the nipple. This allows you to change to the internal jugular approach if necessary. Drape with sterile towels.

Find the mid-point of the clavicle and from a centimetre below with a 21 gauge needle infiltrate local anaesthetic, aspirating as you insert the needle. As you pass below the clavicle turn the needle medially, aiming behind the sternoclavicular joint. This will allow you to localise the subclavian vein. You may need to change to a longer 19 gauge needle at this point.

Having found the vein either take the definitive cannula and insert it down the same tract, or use a larger bore needle and then a guide wire to insert the definitive cannula.

It is often a help to make a 2–3 mm incision at the intended point of insertion to ease the passage of the cannula through the skin.

Finally, secure the cannula with a stitch, spray the entry site with povidone iodine and dress the site. If blood flows easily when you aspirate through the cannula then it is almost certainly in the right place. However, a chest X-ray will be definitive and exclude the very occasional haemo- or pneumothorax.

(2) Internal jugular approach for insertion of central lines

As before explain to the patient what you are going to do, and prepare the same area as described above.

The easier side of approach is the right, so ask the patient to turn his head to the left in a head-down position. If he now lifts his head a fraction off the bed, this displays the apex of the two heads of sternomastoid; allow him to relax back onto the bed. From the apex of this triangle, infiltrate with local anaesthetic, aiming one third of the way between the right nipple and the mid-line and at 45° to the skin. This should allow you to find the internal jugular vein, which can then be cannulated as before.

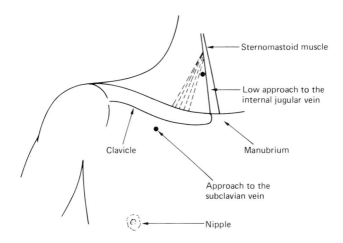

Fig. 11.1 Central line insertion

(3) Radial artery cannulation

This is either performed for sampling blood gases or for the insertion of radial artery pressure lines. Allen's test to confirm that the ulna artery will supply the hand through the palmar arch should be performed (occlude both arteries until the hand becomes pale and then ensure that the hand becomes pink again when the ulna artery is released). Then extend the wrist as far as possible and palpate the artery, localising it 2 cm proximal to the proximal wrist crease. Use a 22 gauge cannula and insert it at an angle of 30° to the skin as if you were inserting a peripheral venous cannula, using the flash back to confirm entry into the artery. Sometimes this is best seen as you withdraw after an apparently failed attempt. If you simply wish to take a radial artery sample, then use a 23 gauge needle on a heparinised syringe and approach the vessel in the same way. After removal of the needle or cannula apply adequate pressure to ensure haemostasis.

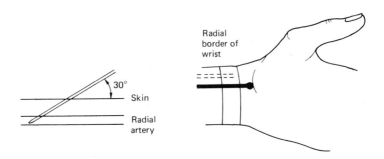

Fig. 11.2 Radial artery cannulation

(4) Insertion of chest drains

Chest drains are inserted because of an accumulation of fluid, gas or both in the pleural space. They should always be inserted from the mid-axillary line, a low insertion point for a haemothorax and a high insertion point for a pneumothorax. It is very rare to require an alternative insertion site.

For a pneumothorax, if possible, sit the patient up at about 30–45°, making sure both that he is comfortable and that you have explained what you are about to do. Make sure that the arm is abducted and supported, follow the second intercostal space around from the manubrio-sternal angle to the mid-axillary line and note the position. Next clean and drape the field in a sterile fashion, and infiltrate with local anaesthetic, use enough to anaesthetise the skin both at the point of insertion and down to and including the pleura. At this time you should be able to aspirate air from the pleural space. If you cannot then either you have not infiltrated far enough or there is not a pneumothorax.

Next choose your drain; for the average male this should be a 24 Ch size; not only do smaller drains tend to kink and obstruct but also the potential flow is proportional to the fourth power of the radius of the tube. Now compare the length of the drain with the patient so that you will insert it an adequate but not excessive distance, its tip should reach the level of the clavicle at the mid-clavicular point.

Now make a 1.5 cm incision horizontally at the point of insertion and place a single vertical mattress suture through it, leaving the ends long with a knot at the end and so that the two ends lie together. (The classical purse string simply turns a straight-line scar into a round puckered messy scar without being any more secure.) Place a single stitch at one end of the incision: this should be '0' nylon at least. Tie this down leaving both ends long as it will be used to secure the drain.

Having done this create a track for the drain by inserting and spreading the point of an artery forceps, which opens up the muscle fibres and should be continued until the forceps opens into the pleural space. Take the drain on its trocar and pass it down the track you have created. Provided the track is adequate it should be possible to do this with the minimum of force and hence risk. Once into the pleural space withdraw the trocar 2 cm and then use it to angle the drain into the correct position and pass the drain over the trocar into the chest. If you have made the skin incision over the 4th rib it will be easier as you pass the drain through the 3rd space to angle the drain correctly.

Connect the drain to an underwater seal bottle, ensuring that it bubbles and swings. Finally secure the drain with the stitch and apply a dressing. Suction is applied if there is a persisting air leak or swing after the drain has been inserted for a pneumothorax; if there is a haemothorax then suction may help to clear it. Usually 5 kPa of suction is applied initially.

Insertion of a drain for haemothorax follows the same procedure, except that you should work your way down from the manubrio-sternal joint to the sixth or seventh space. Use at least a 28 Ch drain, percuss out the collection, aspirate fluid and direct the drain in a more horizontal direction than for a pneumothorax. Finally check a portable chest X-ray to ensure a satisfactory result.

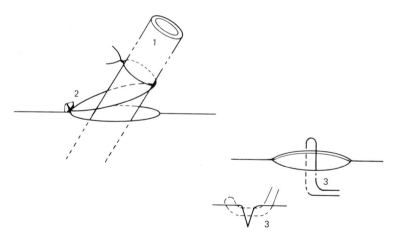

Fig. 11.3 Technique for anchoring Intercostal drains
1   Drain   2   Stitch
3   Single Vertical mattress stitch   (knot to prevent movement at skin)
     for later closure of skin incision.

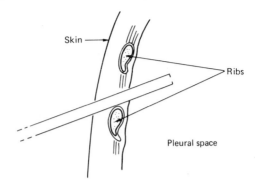

Fig. 11.4   Angled line of insertion of Chest drain

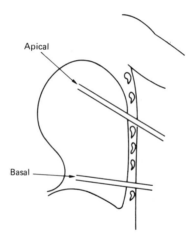

Fig. 11.5   Diagram of chest drain positioning

(5) Suprapubic catheterisation

Failure to pass a urethral catheter suggests the need to insert a suprapubic catheter. This is often much easier, quicker and less damaging than repeated attempts at urethral manipulation. Having explained the procedure to the patient, percuss out the bladder and ensure that it is full. Then prepare and drape the abdomen between the umbilicus and the pubis, staying in the mid-line, infiltrate local anaesthetic down to the bladder and aspirate urine. Using a catheter mounted on a stylette pass it through the anaesthetised area down into the bladder and aspirate urine. Then pass the catheter over the stylette into the bladder, and as the catheter passes into the bladder withdraw the stylette. Finally, connect up the catheter and secure it to the skin.

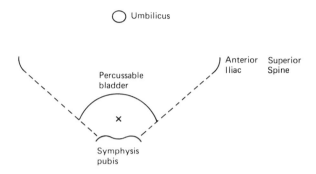

Fig. 11.6 Suprapubic catheterisation

(6) Insertion of flotation pulmonary artery catheter (Swan–Ganz)

This is easier when approached by the internal jugular route, and most units will have available an introducer set which is inserted by the Seldinger technique. This has a valve which allows easy manipulation of the catheter. First explain the procedure to the patient and insert the introducer as described for central venous cannulation. Next remove the cannula from the package and check the balloon, having done this flush all the separate channels with heparinised saline and connect the distal pulmonary artery channel to a pressure monitor, making sure that it will display the pressure waveform. Now pass the polythene catheter guard over the catheter and up it to the proximal end.

With the balloon deflated, pass the catheter through the introducer and when the tip has passed out of the distal end inflate the balloon, whilst watching the pressure tracing smoothly feed the catheter through the introducer. As you advance through the tricuspid valve, the pressure tracing will change to the much more active right ventricular trace, which will show a systolic pressure of around 30 mm Hg and a diastolic of around 0 mm Hg in a normal individual. Now insert the catheter further with 2–3 cm increments, and you should see it pass through the pulmonary valve, at which time the pressure tracing changes to a slightly lower systolic pressure and a markedly higher diastolic pressure, usually around 10 mm

Hg. Still with the balloon up pass the catheter on until it 'wedges'; this is seen by a loss of the dynamic pulmonary artery pressure tracing, and its change to a pressure tracing of about 8 mm Hg that fluctuates slightly with respiration. Deflate the balloon and check that you regain the dynamic pulmonary artery trace, which prevents you over-wedging the catheter. If it remains wedged when you deflate the balloon then withdraw the catheter until you regain the pulmonary artery trace, and then reinflate the balloon and reinsert it as necessary; it should now wedge satisfactorily. Always deflate the balloon when withdrawing the catheter to prevent inadvertent valvular damage. The catheter should never be left in the wedged position and once a measurement has been taken the balloon should be deflated and the catheter withdrawn 2 cm. Often the ability to 'wedge' is lost and then it is usually reasonable to follow the pulmonary artery diastolic pressure.

The protective polythene sheath should then be connected to the introducer so that the catheter can be reinserted the 2–3 cm necessary to take further measurements without compromising the sterility of the system. The catheter should then be firmly secured to the patient, and the pulmonary artery trace displayed to prevent unrecognised accidental 'wedging'.

With a thermodilution catheter you can measure cardiac output. If this is combined with the measurement of right atrial, pulmonary artery, and the pulmonary artery capillary wedge pressures with the catheter and the arterial pressure, then both pulmonary and systemic vascular resistances can be calculated (see Chapter 20).

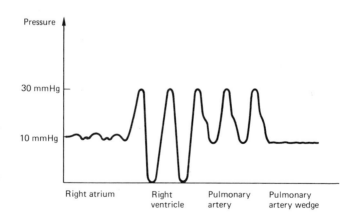

Fig. 11.7   Swan–Ganz insertion pressure trace.

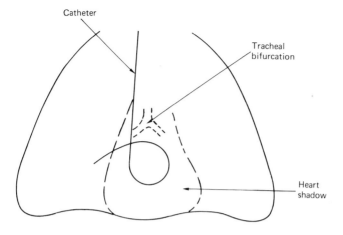

Fig. 11.8 Swan-Ganz catheter positioning on chest x-ray.

(7) Insertion of mini-tracheostomy

This simple procedure for the treatment of sputum retention is frequently lifesaving. The principle is to create a temporary stoma in the crico-thyroid membrane, and through it pass a suction catheter and aspirate the endo-tracheal and endo-bronchial secretions. Whilst most commonly used in thoracic surgery, it can be used at any time that sputum retention alone is a concern. If done correctly it should not impair vocal cord function, nor cause tracheal stricture. It is possible to intubate patients past a mini-tracheostomy but it should then be removed.

Place the patient in a comfortable position with him reclining in bed supported by pillows at about 60°. Extend the neck to throw the laryngeal prominence into view, run your fingers down from the prominence of the thyroid cartilage staying strictly in the mid-line. As your fingers run off the inferior surface of the thyroid cartilage you will feel a slight dip into a space with a slightly elastic feel. Just below this is the hard ring of the cricoid cartilage which you must identify. It is into this space that you will introduce the catheter. Now prepare and drape around this area and infiltrate local anaesthetic around the area you have just identified, making sure that you infiltrate through the membrane. You should now have available a proprietary kit that includes both the catheter and the introducer. With the knife also included make a transverse incision that passes straight down through the skin and through the crico-thyroid membrane. It is much easier if the patient can hold his breath whilst you do this. As soon as you remove the blade insert the introducer through the skin at a perpendicular to the skin, and as it passes through the crico-thyroid membrane turn the introducer so that it slides in an inferior direction into the trachea for 4–5 cm. The catheter will already be mounted on the introducer and it should be gently slid over the introducer which is held firmly until the catheter is partly in the trachea and is then withdrawn as the catheter is fully inserted.

Often at this stage the patient will cough so ensure you hold the catheter securely as he does. (It is worth standing to one side whilst you do this.) Use a fine gauge suction catheter to clear the airway of sputum and any blood, and finally carefully secure the catheter with tapes.

It is possible to jet ventilate through a mini-tracheostomy if this is preferable to (re)intubation.

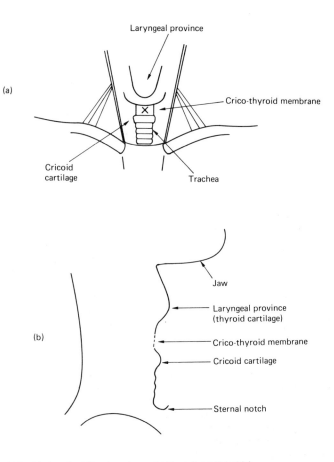

Fig. 11.9 (a) site of mini-tracheostomy; (b) Neck (from the side).

(8) Intra-aortic balloon pumping

The principle of the intra-aortic balloon pump (IABP) is very elegant. Coronary artery blood flow to the left ventricle occurs mainly in diastole. The resistance against which the ventricle contracts (or after-load) governs myocardial energy requirements. The IABP works by inflating in diastole and therefore pushing blood back down the coronary arteries and then deflating in systole. The systolic deflation effectively creates a vacuum which reduces the afterload as the ventricle contracts and therefore reduces the energy requirement of the ventricle. The standard adult balloon inflates to 40 cm^3.

On the radial arterial pressure tracing you will see a peak due to ventricular contraction, and as the aortic valve closes (shown by the dichrotic notch), you will then see the start of the upstroke of the next peak which is generated by the IABP inflating. Finally you will see the peak dip into a trough before the next ventricular systole.

There are several ways of timing the point of IABP inflation; most commonly this is from the 'R' wave of the ECG. It is better if the balloon pump has its own set of ECG leads, though it can be driven off an ECG monitor, from pressure transducers, pacing spikes or a regular internally generated timing mark.

The volume to which the balloon fills (or augmentation) can be adjusted as can the frequency at which it augments, i.e. every cycle or every second or third cycle.

Techniques exist for percutaneous insertion, and also for insertion of the IABP under direct vision, although a skin tunnel technique can also be used. Similarly it is generally removed by the same method by which it was inserted. The patient is heparinised to an ACT of 180–200 from the day after insertion if this occurred after bypass, and from the time of insertion otherwise.

The authors' favoured method in males is to start with a percutaneous technique and if not successful turn to open exposure of the artery and combine that with the percutaneous technique under direct vision. In women open exposure is more often used as the first step due to the frequency of small femoral arteries. Removal at an open procedure is usually combined with passage of an embolectomy catheter and vein patch of the artery. The authors' preference is to use a small balloon catheter without a central lumen to reduce the risk of limb ischaemia, the exception being when it has been necessary to insert the balloon catheter over a guide wire. The position of the balloon catheter should be checked on a CXR: the tip should lie alongside the 5th thoracic vertebra.

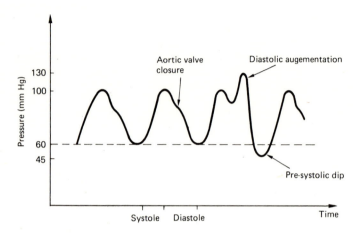

Fig. 11.10   Schematic intra-aortic balloon pump trace.

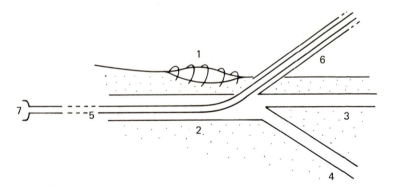

Fig. 11.11   Direct vision 'percutaneous' approach.
1   Skin incision   2   Common femoral artery
3   Superficial femoral artery   4   Profunda femoral artery
5   Balloon catheter   6   Sheath (withdrawn)
7   Balloon

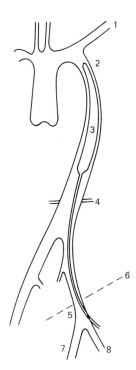

Fig. 11.12   Positioning of intra-aortic balloon pump.
 1 Left subclavian artery   2 Radio opaque marker
 3 Balloon   4 Renal arteries
 5 Common femoral artery   6 Line of inguinal ligament
 7 Superficial femoral artery   8 Profunda femoral artery

(9) Haemofiltration

The technique of haemofiltration is becoming of increasing use on the ICU. It is a simple method of treating moderate to severe renal failure. The technique comprises continuous arterio-venous or veno-venous ultra-filtration across a small membrane that is highly permeable to water. Electrolytes and small and medium-sized molecules (less than 50 000 daltons) are filtered, the process being driven either by arterial pressure in the arterio-venous form or by a small pump in the veno-venous form. Simultaneously the blood volume can, if necessary, be reconstituted by the infusion of an electrolyte solution that approximates to normal plasma, though with variations according to the clinical needs.

As indicated above, there are two different modifications to the technique. In the first a cannula must be placed into the femoral artery for blood supply into the filter and a second into the femoral vein for the return of blood to the circulation. This has the risk of damage to the femoral artery. The authors' preference is to insert a double lumen catheter into either the subclavian or internal jugular vein. This has the advantage of a single vascular puncture site, it is more comfortable than the femoral site and as there is less movement, it is easier to prevent infection at the puncture site. It has the minor drawback of requiring a small pump to maintain flow.

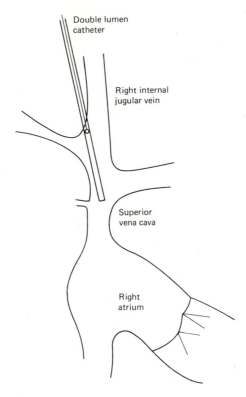

Fig. 11.13 Haemofiltration using double lumen catheter.

The aim is to provide renal replacement therapy and as such it has two functions. Firstly if it is solely necessary to remove excess blood volume alone then only relatively small volumes need to be taken off. As an example, taking off 100 ml/h will provide an 'output' of 2.4l per 24 hours. If treatment of biochemical abnormalities is required, then the volume taken off can be increased, in practice up to 1 l/h can be taken off. If this is replaced with 900 ml/h of a proprietary haemofiltration solution, then not only will the patient's biochemistry be improved, but also a negative balance can be achieved if this is desired.

If it proves difficult to take off adequate volume, then there are various manoeuvres that can be tried, including applying a few kilopascals of suction to the filtrate side of the filter or applying a gate clamp to the venous side and *partially* occluding the venous line. Each manoeuvre increases the pressure across the membrane.

It is usual to heparinise the patient to an ACT of 160–180 to prevent the filter clotting.

(10) Continuous haemodialysis (haemodiafiltration)

Continuous haemodialysis is a newer technique, derived from a combination of haemofiltration and intermittent haemodialysis. Like haemofiltration it can be run as either an arterio-venous or veno-venous technique. It has the advantage of requiring lower volumes of fluid replacement and of blood flow through the filter.

The haemofiltration type coil is modified so that an electrolyte solution can be run in a counter current direction to the blood stream across the membrane. This allows both the removal of fluid by ultrafiltration and also the dialysis of permeable molecules across the membrane down the concentration gradient.

Generally the flow of dialysis fluid is less than 1 l/h, and this allows full equilibration across the membrane whilst the low blood flow avoids gross haemodynamic instability.

The dialysate can be PD fluid, haemofiltration solution or other fluids according to the clinical requirement.

The cannulation technique is identical to that of haemofiltration and heparinisation to an ACT of 180 s is required.

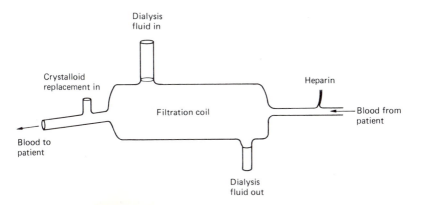

Fig. 11.14 Continuous haemodialysis circuit.

(11) D.C. cardioversion

D.C. cardioversion is indicated for the control of life threatening arrhythmias, as well as the control of arrhythmias resistant to medical treatment. As it can be very uncomfortable the patient should be sedated before emergency cardioversion and anaesthetised before elective cardioversion.

One paddle should be placed over the middle of the sternum, in the mid-line. The second paddle should be placed just lateral to the apex, usually on the anterior axillary line. Conducting pads or jelly must completely cover the skin under the paddles.

The defibrillator should then be charged to the required energy. For supraventricular arrhythmias, start at around 0.5 to 0.75 J/kg, for ventricular tachycardia or fibrillation start at around 1.5 J/kg and increase if it is not possible to control the arrhythmia. The maximum energy that can be delivered to an adult by a defibrillator is around 4–5 J/kg; for a child the maximum energy used is around 5 J/kg.

In ventricular fibrillation it is not necessary to use the synchronised mode; however, it should be used for other arrhythmias to prevent the induction of ventricular fibrillation by accident.

If the patient suffers burns from the paddles, then topical hydrocortisone cream should be applied.

Always ensure that all staff are clear of the patient and not in contact with any potential electrically conducting structure attached to the patient. Pacing boxes should be switched off when the shock is given.

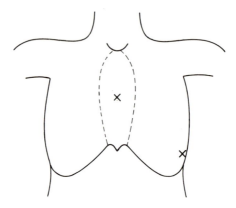

Fig. 11.15 Paddle sites for d.c. cardioversion.

Part 2

The aim of this part of the handbook is to provide an 'on the spot' guide to the management of problems that will worry the inexperienced ICU resident or nurse who is facing a new and often difficult environment.

Various conditions will be discussed in a problem-orientated manner, and the pathways by which the management decisions are made will be demonstrated by flow diagrams. Whilst these pathways might look rigid, they are designed to show a safe though not necessarily unique line of approach.

At the end of the book will be found a series of lists of normal values, together with drug data that will help both in the assessment and management of these problems.

Remember, if in doubt, take senior advice.

12
Post-operative hypotension

The easiest guide to management of post-operative hypotension is the central venous pressure (CVP).

(1)

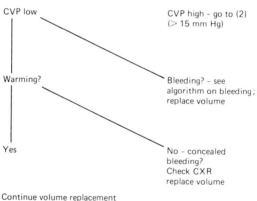

CVP low   CVP high - go to (2)
(> 15 mm Hg)

Warming?   Bleeding? – see
algorithm on bleeding;
replace volume

Yes   No - concealed
bleeding?
Check CXR
replace volume

Continue volume replacement
Check CXR if over 750 ml + balance

(2)

CVP High: There are spurious causes for a raised CVP, including; high zero, kinked and/or partially obstructed lines, concurrent drug administration through the line, the patient trying to breathe against the ventilator or the use of PEEP by the anaesthetist. If in doubt always check the pressure trace on a monitor or look at the swing on a simple manometer.

The question that needs answering is: is this pump failure or is it tamponade?

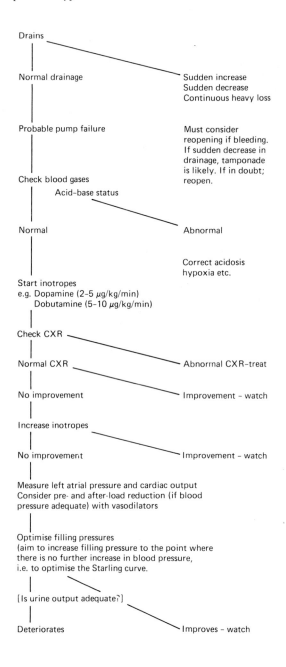

Drains

Normal drainage

Sudden increase
Sudden decrease
Continuous heavy loss

Probable pump failure

Must consider
reopening if bleeding.
If sudden decrease in
drainage, tamponade
is likely. If in doubt;
reopen.

Check blood gases
          Acid–base status

Normal

Abnormal

Correct acidosis
hypoxia etc.

Start inotropes
e.g. Dopamine (2–5 µg/kg/min)
     Dobutamine (5–10 µg/kg/min)

Check CXR

Normal CXR

Abnormal CXR-treat

No improvement

Improvement – watch

Increase inotropes

No improvement

Improvement – watch

Measure left atrial pressure and cardiac output
Consider pre- and after-load reduction (if blood
pressure adequate) with vasodilators

Optimise filling pressures
(aim to increase filling pressure to the point where
there is no further increase in blood pressure,
i.e. to optimise the Starling curve.

[Is urine output adequate?]

Deteriorates

Improves – watch

At this stage you will probably be using maximal doses of inotropes such as dopamine (10 μg/kg/min) and dobutamine (10–15 μg/kg/min), it is now worth changing to adrenaline as the inotrope of choice and continuing with a renal dose of dopamine. It would have been quite reasonable to have started with dopamine and added adrenaline as the second inotrope earlier, particularly if problems had been expected.

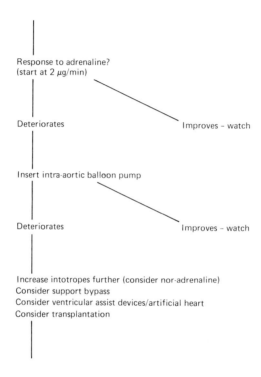

Although the insertion of the IABP has been quite late in the sequence as shown, it may be appropriate to insert it earlier in the high-risk patient in whom problems are expected. If it has proved difficult or impossible to wean from bypass, then its use will have started in theatre; the advantage of this is that it can be inserted quickly and easily in theatre under sterile conditions.

The criterion for left ventricular assistance is a technically successful open heart procedure with subsequent refractory cardiogenic shock. This is defined by a mean left atrial pressure greater than 25 mm Hg with a systolic arterial pressure less than 90 mm Hg and a cardiac index of less than 1.6 l/min/M2. The indications for right entricular assistance are similar with a mean right atrial pressure (in the absence of tricuspid regurgitation) greater than 25 mm Hg, a low left atrial pressure and a cardiac index of less than 1.6 l/min/M2.

13
Post-operative hypertension

It is important to control hypertension in the early post-operative period, most importantly afterload is increased and hence the work performed by the heart during a potentially unstable period. Bleeding is more likely and will be more profuse in the hypertensive patient. It will also be more difficult to warm up the patient while he is intensely vasoconstricted. The following algorithm is a strategy for the management of early post-operative hypertension. Once the patient has returned to the ward then simple measures such as oral vasodilators and beta blockers will usually be quite adequate.

Hypertension
(systolic > 120 mm Hg, or mean > 85 mm Hg)

(1)

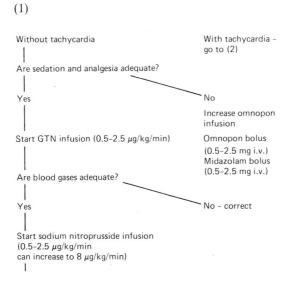

Without tachycardia
|
Are sedation and analgesia adequate?
|
Yes
|
Start GTN infusion (0.5–2.5 μg/kg/min)
|
Are blood gases adequate?
|
Yes
|
Start sodium nitroprusside infusion
(0.5–2.5 μg/kg/min
can increase to 8 μg/kg/min)
|

With tachycardia –
go to (2)

No

Increase omnopon
infusion
Omnopon bolus
(0.5–2.5 mg i.v.)
Midazolam bolus
(0.5–2.5 mg i.v.)

No – correct

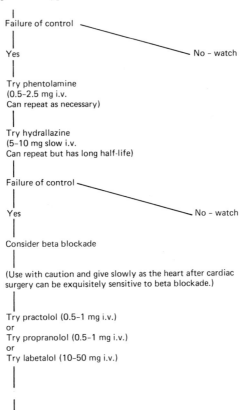

Failure of control

Yes ——————————————— No – watch

Try phentolamine
(0.5–2.5 mg i.v.
Can repeat as necessary)

Try hydrallazine
(5–10 mg slow i.v.
Can repeat but has long half-life)

Failure of control

Yes ——————————————— No – watch

Consider beta blockade

(Use with caution and give slowly as the heart after cardiac surgery can be exquisitely sensitive to beta blockade.)

Try practolol (0.5–1 mg i.v.)
or
Try propranolol (0.5–1 mg i.v.)
or
Try labetalol (10–50 mg i.v.)

In general if there is an episode of rebound hypotension, then it can be treated by rapid volume replacement and the discontinuation of the vasodilator infusions. If this proves unsuccessful then a bolus of calcium chloride (5–10 mmol i.v.) is usually effective; alternatives include phenylephrine, metariminol or adrenaline.

(2)

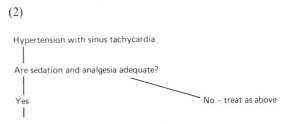

Hypertension with sinus tachycardia

Are sedation and analgesia adequate?

Yes ——————————————— No – treat as above

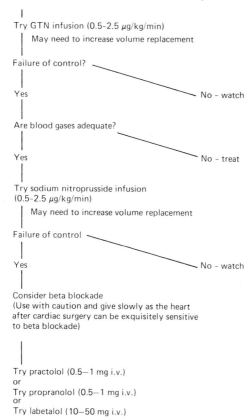

Try GTN infusion (0.5-2.5 µg/kg/min)
   May need to increase volume replacement

Failure of control?

Yes   No – watch

Are blood gases adequate?

Yes   No – treat

Try sodium nitroprusside infusion
(0.5-2.5 µg/kg/min)
   May need to increase volume replacement

Failure of control

Yes   No – watch

Consider beta blockade
(Use with caution and give slowly as the heart
after cardiac surgery can be exquisitely sensitive
to beta blockade)

Try practolol (0.5–1 mg i.v.)
or
Try propranolol (0.5–1 mg i.v.)
or
Try labetalol (10–50 mg i.v.)

If tachycardia is a problem then the other intravenous vasodilators are relatively contra-indicated; if rebound hypotension occurs then it can be treated with volume replacement and if necessary calcium chloride (5–10 mmol i.v.) or vasopressor agents.

14

Post-operative bleeding

Bleeding in the early post-operative period may be catastrophic and it can be one of the most stressful events to occur on the ICU. In the event of a sudden, massive bleed *do not hesitate:* whilst other people get help, *reopen* the patient, *control the bleeding point* and then wait for help. Whilst sucking out the blood and clot may help to find the site of bleeding, as soon as possible control the bleeding point, with a finger or a clamp as necessary and try to avoid further loss of blood until the patient's blood pressure has been controlled.

Possible bleeding points include; aortic cannulation sites, aortomy and cardioplegia sites, vent sites, proximal and distal vein graft anastomoses, side branches on vein or internal mammary artery, atrial cannulation and atriotomy sites.

Severe bleeding, more than 400 ml/h usually requires urgent re-exploration, preferably in the operating theatre. The algorithm that follows discusses the management of patients that fall into the moderate (under 200 ml/h) and heavy (200–400 ml/h) groups.

Always be sure to have adequate supplies of blood in the same place as the patients, be it the ICU or the operating theatre. If tamponade is suspected then it is better to re-explore early rather than (too) late. Tamponade can occur when one or even both pleural cavities are open; under these circumstances it is both harder to diagnose and slower to be recognised.

Is the bleeding moderate or heavy (as defined above)?

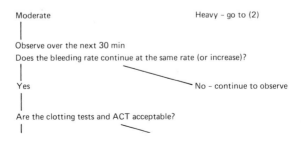

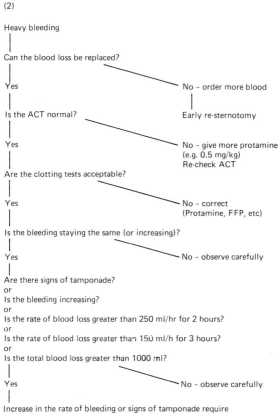

Yes | No – correct
(Protamine, FFP, etc.)

Is the bleeding increasing?
or
Is the bleeding more than
150 ml/h for 3 hours
or
1000 ml in total?

Yes | No – observe

Consider re-sternotomy

(2)

Heavy bleeding

Can the blood loss be replaced?

Yes | No – order more blood

Is the ACT normal? | Early re-sternotomy

Yes | No – give more protamine
(e.g. 0.5 mg/kg)
Re-check ACT

Are the clotting tests acceptable?

Yes | No – correct
(Protamine, FFP, etc)

Is the bleeding staying the same (or increasing)?

Yes | No – observe carefully

Are there signs of tamponade?
or
Is the bleeding increasing?
or
Is the rate of blood loss greater than 250 ml/hr for 2 hours?
or
Is the rate of blood loss greater than 150 ml/h for 3 hours?
or
Is the total blood loss greater than 1000 ml?

Yes | No – observe carefully

Increase in the rate of bleeding or signs of tamponade require
immediate re-sternotomy; an unacceptable rate of bleeding or
total amount of blood loss suggest the need for early
re-sternotomy.

15
Post-operative arrhythmias

In the management of post-operative arrhythmias there are two important points to be considered; firstly, is the cardiac output maintained and secondly, is there a precipitating factor for the development of the arrhythmia? The degree of urgency in the treatment of an arrhythmia depends on its haemodynamic effects. The development of ventricular fibrillation requires immediate cardiac massage and d.c. cardioversion. The onset of controlled atrial fibrillation may be investigated before treatment is started in most cases.

Precipitating factors for the development of post-operative arrhythmias include hypokalaemia, hypoxia, hypercarbia, pericardial collections, pulmonary collapse and even toxic digoxin levels (after redistribution by bypass). Whilst not specifically mentioned in the following series of algorithms, the chest should always be examined at the earliest possible moment and the ventilator functions checked. If in doubt it is always safer to switch to manual ventilation on 100% oxygen.

Don't try to cardiovert a patient who is still awake – it is a frightening and painful experience – and always ensure that everyone is away from the patient when the d.c. shock is given.

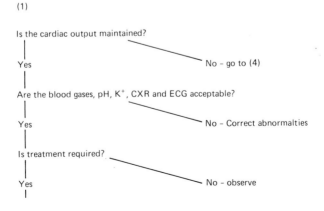

(1)

Is the cardiac output maintained?

Yes   No – go to (4)

Are the blood gases, pH, K^+, CXR and ECG acceptable?

Yes   No – Correct abnormalties

Is treatment required?

Yes   No – observe

Bradyarrythmia or tachyarrythmia?

Bradyarrythmia   Tachyarrythmia – go to (3)

Is it nodal rhythm?

No   Yes – go to (2)

Is a pacing wire present?

Yes   No – try atropine (0.3-0.6 mg)
                                                 — Try isoprenaline
                                                    (0.1–0.25 mg)
                                                 — try isoprenaline infusion
Pace   — insert pacing wire

(2)

Nodal rhythm

Try CaCl (5–10 mmol)
     Atropine (0.3–1.2 mg)
     Isoprenaline (0.1–0.25 mg)
     Atrial pacing
     A-V sequential pacing

(3)

Tachyarrythmias

Is the K^+ above 4.5 mmol/l?

Yes   No – treat
                                                 (e.g. 0.1-0.2 mmol/kg of K^+)

Is the arrythmia atrial or ventricular?

Atrial   Ventricular
- try digoxin (0.75 mg/M2 total)   - try lignocaine (25-50 mg)
  (give in 0.125 mg increments   and/or infusion
or   or
- try verapamil (2.5-6 mg)   - try amiodarone
or   (300 mg in 3 hours then
- try practolol (0.5-2.5 mg)   900 mg in 21 hours)
or   or
- try amiodarone   - D.C.cardioversion
  (300 mg in 20 min to 3 h then
  900 mg in 21 hours)

(4)

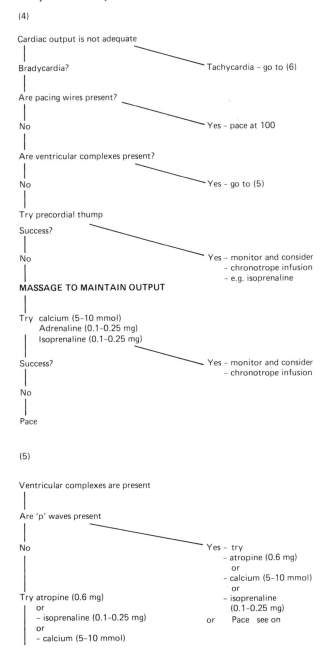

Cardiac output is not adequate

Bradycardia? ——————————→ Tachycardia – go to (6)

Are pacing wires present? —————→ Yes – pace at 100

No

Are ventricular complexes present? ——→ Yes – go to (5)

No

Try precordial thump
Success? ——————————————→ Yes – monitor and consider
                                       – chronotrope infusion
No   – e.g. isoprenaline

MASSAGE TO MAINTAIN OUTPUT

Try calcium (5–10 mmol)
      Adrenaline (0.1–0.25 mg)
      Isoprenaline (0.1–0.25 mg)

Success? ——————————————→ Yes – monitor and consider
                                       – chronotrope infusion
No

Pace

(5)

Ventricular complexes are present

Are 'p' waves present ——————————→ Yes – try
                                          – atropine (0.6 mg)
No   or
                                          – calcium (5–10 mmol)
                                            or
                                          – isoprenaline
                                            (0.1–0.25 mg)
Try atropine (0.6 mg)   or   Pace see on
      or
      – isoprenaline (0.1–0.25 mg)
      or
      – calcium (5–10 mmol)

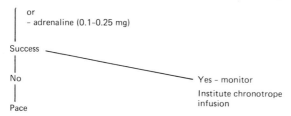

or
– adrenaline (0.1–0.25 mg)

Success

No   Yes – monitor
                                      Institute chronotrope
Pace   infusion

Pacing

If epicardial wires have been left on at the time of operation then use them. If epicardial wires are not available, or are not working, then there are various other strategies. These range from inserting temporary endocardial wires through a transvenous approach, through oesophageal or even transcutaneous stimulation to reopening the chest and applying epicardial wires. In practical terms the choice will lie between a transvenous approach and reopening the chest.

There are a variety of transvenous wires available ranging from the simple 'temporary' wire to balloon flotation pacing catheters and specific wires designed to pace the atrium – the 'J' wires.
(6)

Tachyarrhythmias

Most of these require treatment. If the cardiac output is severely compromised, then massage is required to maintain the output. Often there is a 'grey area' where treatment is required urgently but immediate defibrillation is not necessary but is required after the failure of first-line medical treatment. If the output becomes severely compromised then immediate defibrillation becomes the therapy of choice.

Whilst resuscitation is being instituted, make arrangements to check the serum potassium, the blood gases and acid-base status, ensure that the patient is adequately ventilated.

Atrial   Ventricular – go to (7)

Try verapamil (up to 10 mg)
     or
     – digoxin (up to 1.5 mg [give as repeated 0.125 mg boluses])
     or
     disopyramide (50–100 mg)
     or
     – amiodarone (300 mg over 20 min to 3 hours)

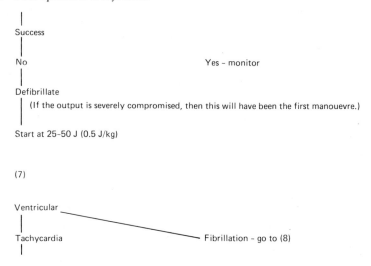

|
Success
|
No   Yes – monitor
|
Defibrillate
| (If the output is severely compromised, then this will have been the first manouevre.)
|
Start at 25-50 J (0.5 J/kg)

(7)

Ventricular
|
Tachycardia ———————————————→ Fibrillation – go to (8)
|

Ventricular tachycardia occasionally occurs as a single episode that is of short duration (less than 10 complexes) and self-terminating, in these cases it is usually adequate to check that the potassium and gases are adequate and monitor the patient. If there are more than 10 complexes, more than one episode or frequent or multi-focal ectopics then 50–100 mg of lignocaine should be given.

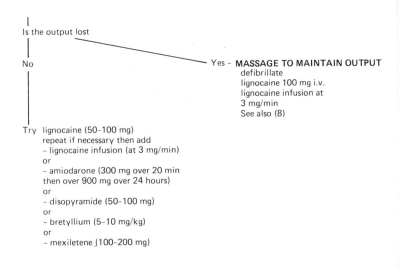

|
Is the output lost
|
No   Yes – **MASSAGE TO MAINTAIN OUTPUT**
| defibrillate
| lignocaine 100 mg i.v.
| lignocaine infusion at
| 3 mg/min
| See also (8)
|
Try lignocaine (50-100 mg)
     repeat if necessary then add
     – lignocaine infusion (at 3 mg/min)
     or
     – amiodarone (300 mg over 20 min
     then over 900 mg over 24 hours)
     or
     – disopyramide (50-100 mg)
     or
     – bretyllium (5-10 mg/kg)
     or
     – mexiletene (100-200 mg)

Failure to control the tachycardia at any time or the loss of output are indications to proceed to d.c. cardioversion. In some cases overdrive pacing can be used in the control of ventricular tachycardia.

(8)

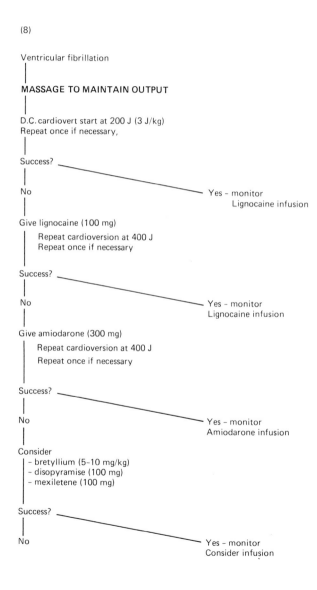

Ventricular fibrillation

MASSAGE TO MAINTAIN OUTPUT

D.C. cardiovert start at 200 J (3 J/kg)
Repeat once if necessary,

Success?

No   Yes – monitor
                 Lignocaine infusion

Give lignocaine (100 mg)
    Repeat cardioversion at 400 J
    Repeat once if necessary

Success?

No   Yes – monitor
                 Lignocaine infusion

Give amiodarone (300 mg)
    Repeat cardioversion at 400 J
    Repeat once if necessary

Success?

No   Yes – monitor
                 Amiodarone infusion

Consider
    – bretyllium (5–10 mg/kg)
    – disopyramise (100 mg)
    – mexiletene (100 mg)

Success?

No   Yes – monitor
                 Consider infusion

Certainly at this point, if not before, a decision needs to be taken as to whether the chest should be reopened, as the alternative is probably to abandon attempts at resuscitation at this stage. It is always possible to continue from here but it is probable that some form of support bypass will be required if the patient is to survive. Reopening the chest will allow an assessment to be made of graft patency in coronary artery grafting and valve function in valve surgery.

(9) Ventricular premature beats

Ventricular premature beats are common but less dramatic; however, they may precede a deterioration into a more unstable rhythm. The potassium should be maintained at 4.5–5.0 mmol/l and if this fails to abolish the VPBs then treatment with lignocaine should be considered (see 7).

16
Impaired gas exchange

Early post-operative respiratory dysfunction will present as either abnormal blood gas measurements, or as cardiovascular instability. Obviously, therefore, in the presence of cardiovascular instability one should check both the gases and serum potassium early in the course of resuscitation.

This section is designed to help in the management and treatment of respiratory dysfunction in the post-operative period.

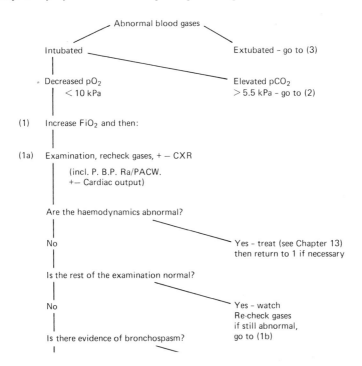

```
         |
        No                          Yes – treat
                                    salbutamol nebulisers
                                      + – aminophylline;
                                    (125–250 mg i.v. bolus
                                    0.5 mg/kg h infusion)


(1b)   Is the CXR normal (if not previously checked)?

         |
       Abnormal
                                    Normal – watch
                                    Repeat gases
                                    – if pO₂ still low;
                                    – increase FiO₂ + – PEEP


       Localised abnormalities      General abnormalities

       Pneumothorax – drain         Pulmonary oedema – treat
       Haemothorax – drain          – diuretics
       Lobar collapse               – vasodilators
       Physiotherapy                – Inotropes
       Bronchoscopy                 – PEEP
       PEEP/CPAP                    – Haemofiltration
        + – antibiotics


(2)    Elevated pCO₂
         |
       Check inflation pressures
         |
       Low                          High – go to (2b)
         |
(2a)   Check patient to ventilator connections

       Connected                    Disconnected –
         |                          – hand bag
         |                          – re-connect.
       Check ventilator parameters
         |
       Correct                      Incorrect –
         |                          – change
         |                          – repeat gases
(2b)   Check tube patency
         |
       Patent                       Impatent

                                    – sputum:   suction
                                                physio
                                    – biting tube;
                                        paralyse change to naso-tracheal
                                        extubate
                                    – kinked tube:
                                        shorten tube
                                        change tube
                                        extubate
                                    – other: in doubt – change tube
```

In the mathematical/chemical notation: pO_2, FiO_2, pCO_2.

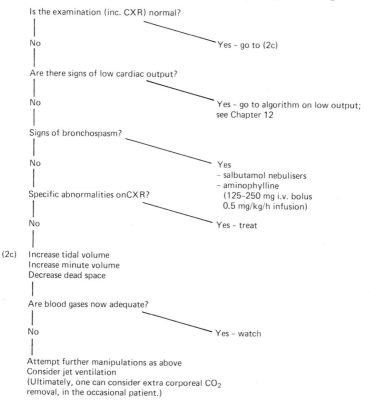

Is the examination (inc. CXR) normal?

No   Yes – go to (2c)

Are there signs of low cardiac output?

No   Yes – go to algorithm on low output; see Chapter 12

Signs of bronchospasm?

No   Yes
                              – salbutamol nebulisers
                              – aminophylline

Specific abnormalities onCXR?   (125–250 mg i.v. bolus
                                  0.5 mg/kg/h infusion)

No   Yes – treat

(2c) Increase tidal volume
       Increase minute volume
       Decrease dead space

Are blood gases now adequate?

No   Yes – watch

Attempt further manipulations as above
Consider jet ventilation
(Ultimately, one can consider extra corporeal CO_2
removal, in the occasional patient.)

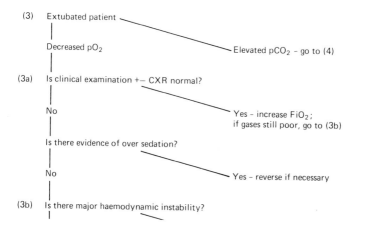

(3)   Extubated patient

Decreased pO_2 Elevated pCO_2 – go to (4)

(3a) Is clinical examination +– CXR normal?

No   Yes – increase FiO_2;
                              if gases still poor, go to (3b)

Is there evidence of over sedation?

No   Yes – reverse if necessary

(3b) Is there major haemodynamic instability?

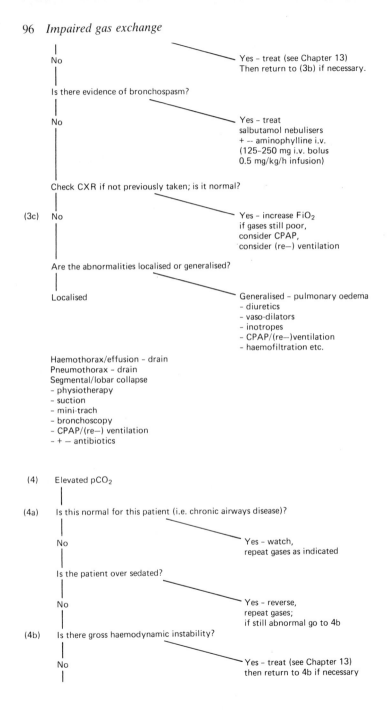

No
Yes – treat (see Chapter 13)
Then return to (3b) if necessary.

Is there evidence of bronchospasm?

No
Yes – treat
salbutamol nebulisers
+ – aminophylline i.v.
(125–250 mg i.v. bolus
0.5 mg/kg/h infusion)

Check CXR if not previously taken; is it normal?

(3c) No
Yes – increase FiO_2
if gases still poor,
consider CPAP,
consider (re–) ventilation

Are the abnormalities localised or generalised?

Localised
Generalised – pulmonary oedema
  – diuretics
  – vaso-dilators
  – inotropes
  – CPAP/(re–)ventilation
  – haemofiltration etc.

Haemothorax/effusion – drain
Pneumothorax – drain
Segmental/lobar collapse
– physiotherapy
– suction
– mini-trach
– bronchoscopy
– CPAP/(re–) ventilation
– + – antibiotics

(4) Elevated pCO_2

(4a) Is this normal for this patient (i.e. chronic airways disease)?

No
Yes – watch,
repeat gases as indicated

Is the patient over sedated?

No
Yes – reverse,
repeat gases;
if still abnormal go to 4b

(4b) Is there gross haemodynamic instability?

No
Yes – treat (see Chapter 13)
then return to 4b if necessary

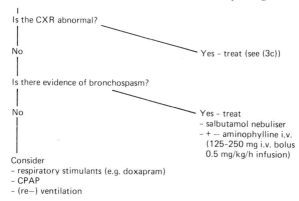

```
|
Is the CXR abnormal?
|
|
No                                    Yes – treat (see (3c))
|
|
Is there evidence of bronchospasm?
|
|
No                                    Yes – treat
|                                     – salbutamol nebuliser
|                                     – + – aminophylline i.v.
|                                       (125-250 mg i.v. bolus
|                                        0.5 mg/kg/h infusion)
Consider
- respiratory stimulants (e.g. doxapram)
- CPAP
- (re–) ventilation
```

The adult respiratory distress syndrome (ARDS) as defined by

$PaO_2 < 50$ mm Hg with FiO_2 40%
PEEP of 5 cm H_2O
New bilateral pulmonary infiltrates
PACW $< = 18$ mm Hg
Normal plasma oncotic pressure

is the more severe end of a spectrum that starts from the so-called 'acute lung injury' sometimes seen after cardiopulmonary bypass. It is a multi-system illness, and its treatment requires support of the cardiac, renal, and metabolic systems in addition to the various forms of respiratory management. There are two main approaches to the management of ARDS at the present time. In one approach the emphasis lies on aggressive diuresis with haemofiltration as required. Cardiac output is supported with the use of inotropes and vasoconstrictors. The second line of approach is to optimise cardiac output with volume loading and inotropes, with frequent assessment of cardiac output and oxygen uptake and delivery.

17
Oliguria and anuria

Elsewhere the arguments against routine urethral catheterisation have been enumerated; however, if there is doubt about the haemodynamic stability of a patient, and in particular if there is a requirement for inotropic support, then catheterisation is necessary. A fall in urine output in the early post-operative period is generally a reflection of either poor cardiac output or simply an inadequate fluid replacement therapy. The algorithm given here suggests a line of management that can be used for post-operative oliguria.

Is the urine output less than 0.5 ml per kg per hour for 2 hours or less than 0.25 ml per kg per hour in any one hour?

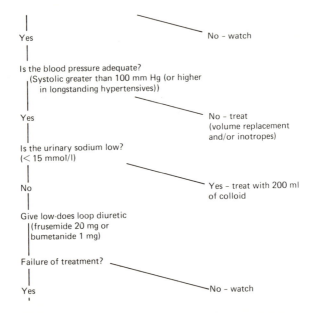

Yes | No – watch

Is the blood pressure adequate?
(Systolic greater than 100 mm Hg (or higher in longstanding hypertensives))

Yes | No – treat
(volume replacement and/or inotropes)

Is the urinary sodium low?
(< 15 mmol/l)

No | Yes – treat with 200 ml of colloid

Give low-does loop diuretic
(frusemide 20 mg or bumetanide 1 mg)

Failure of treatment?

Yes | No – watch

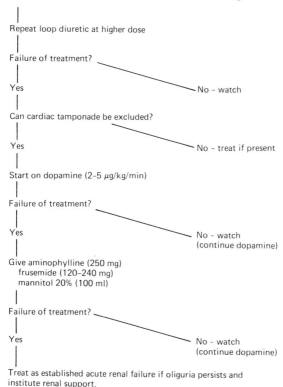

Repeat loop diuretic at higher dose

Failure of treatment?

Yes — No – watch

Can cardiac tamponade be excluded?

Yes — No – treat if present

Start on dopamine (2–5 µg/kg/min)

Failure of treatment?

Yes — No – watch (continue dopamine)

Give aminophylline (250 mg)
frusemide (120–240 mg)
mannitol 20% (100 ml)

Failure of treatment?

Yes — No – watch (continue dopamine)

Treat as established acute renal failure if oliguria persists and institute renal support.

Occasionally an infusion of a potent loop diuretic such as frusemide 500 mg over 4 hours may be effective if established acute renal failure has not occurred; alternatively, ethacrynic acid is sometimes effective when frusemide or bumetanide have failed. If it is necessary to institute haemofiltration in a unit that is not experienced in its management, then advice should be sought from the local renal unit.

Alternatives include continuous arterio-venous (or pumped veno-venous) haemodialysis or peritoneal dialysis.

18
Agitation

The agitated patient can be one of the most difficult to manage, and in the presence of confusion and agitation a series of questions need to be answered. As always the most important relate to cardiac output and the adequacy of ventilation. The management plan given below suggests an approach to the agitated patient and the series of questions that must be answered before a patient is 'just' sedated.

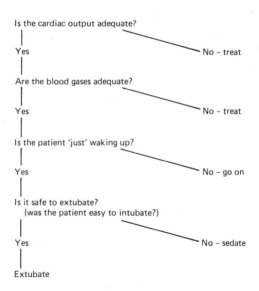

At this point, in both the extubated patient and in the intubated, a further series of questions need to be asked:

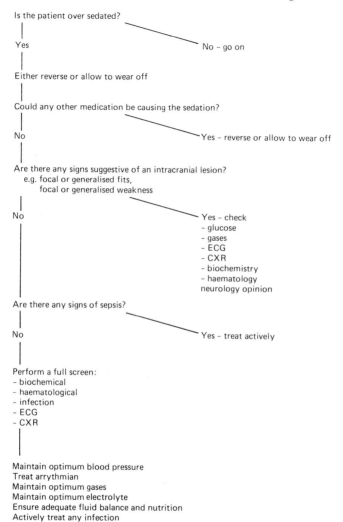

Is the patient over sedated?

Yes   No – go on

Either reverse or allow to wear off

Could any other medication be causing the sedation?

No   Yes – reverse or allow to wear off

Are there any signs suggestive of an intracranial lesion?
 e.g. focal or generalised fits,
   focal or generalised weakness

No   Yes – check
           – glucose
           – gases
           – ECG
           – CXR
           – biochemistry
           – haematology
           neurology opinion

Are there any signs of sepsis?

No   Yes – treat actively

Perform a full screen:
– biochemical
– haematological
– infection
– ECG
– CXR

Maintain optimum blood pressure
Treat arrythmian
Maintain optimum gases
Maintain optimum electrolyte
Ensure adequate fluid balance and nutrition
Actively treat any infection

Obtain neurology opinion with a view to further investigation (CT scan or NMR scan then lumbar puncture if signs of sub-arterial haemorrhage or meningitis).

Part 3

The aim of this part of the handbook is to provide ready access to normal physiological data, together with pharmacological data and infusion tables.

19
Normal values (in adults)

Arterial blood pressures

Systolic 110–130 mm Hg
Diastolic 70–90 mm Hg
Mean   80–100 mm Hg

Left ventricular pressures

Systolic 110–130 mm Hg
End diastolic; before 'a' up to 7 mm Hg on 'a' up to 12 mm Hg

Left atrial pressures

Systolic: 'a' up to 12 mm Hg 'v' up to 10 mm Hg
Diastolic: 'x' up to 7 mm Hg 'y' up to 7 mm Hg
Mean: up to 10 mm Hg

Pulmonary artery pressures

Systolic: up to 25 mm Hg
Diastolic: up to 15 mm Hg
Mean: up to 18 mm Hg
Capillary wedge: mean 10 mm Hg (as for left atrial pressures)

Right ventricular pressures

Systolic: up to 25 mm Hg
End diastolic: before 'a'; up to 3 mm Hg
                On 'a' up to 7 mm Hg

Right atrial pressures

Systolic: 'a' up to 7 mm Hg 'v' up to 5 mm Hg
Diastolic: 'x' up to 3 mm Hg 'y' up to 3 mm Hg
Mean: up to 5 mm Hg

Heart rate 60–90 bpm

P–R interval: 0.12–0.2 s
QRS duration: 0.08–0.1 s
QT interval: 0.40–0.43 s

Cardiac output at rest 5.5 l/min
Cardiac index   at rest 3.2 l/min

Stroke volume   75–80 ml at rest

End systolic volume 50 ml
End diastolic volume 125–135 ml

Calculation of pulmonary vascular resistance

$$\frac{\text{mean pulmonary arterial pressure} - \text{mean left atrial pressure}}{\text{pulmonary blood flow}}$$

Calculation of systemic vascular resistance

$$\frac{\text{mean aortic pressure} - \text{mean right atrial pressure}}{\text{systemic blood flow}}$$

In the absence of significant shunts, the systemic and pulmonary blood flows can be considered to be the same for the purpose of these calculations.

Normal SVR   12–16 (Wood units)
            ($\times$ 80 for dynes s cm^{-5})

Normal PVR Less than 2.5 (Wood units)
            ($\times$ 80 for dynes s cm^{-5})

Quick estimation of left to right shunt
            (e.g. in ischaemic VSD)

$$\frac{\text{aortic saturation} - \text{right atrial saturation}}{\text{aortic saturation} - \text{pulmonary artery saturation}}$$

Normal blood gases

Arterial pO_2: 80–110 mm Hg, 10.5–15 kPa
Arterial pCO_2: 37–42 mm Hg, 5–5.5 kPa
Arterial pH: 7.36–7.44

O_2 saturation: arterial 96–98%
                 Mixed venous 75%

Lung volumes

Tidal volume 500 ml
Dead space   150 ml
Vital capacity 3.1–4.8 l

FEV 1 85% of FVC (forced vital capacity)
Peak flow 450–650 l/min

Normal values in blood

Haematology

	Men		Women
Hb	13.5–17.5		11.5–15.5 gm/dl
WCC		4.0–11.0 '000/mmm	
Platelets		140–400 '000/mmm	
PCV	0.4–0.54		0.37–0.47
MCV		80–90 fl	
Total blood volume		60–80 ml/kg	
Red cell volume	25–35		20–30 ml/kg
Plasma volume		40–50 ml/kg	

Biochemistry

Sodium	135–145 mmol/l
Potassium	3.5–5.0 mmol/l
Chloride	100–106 mmol/l
Bicarbonate	21–27 mmol/l
Urea	3–9 mmol/l
Creatinine	60–130 umol/l
Glucose	3.3–5.6 mmol/l (fasting)
Calcium	2.1–2.6 mmol/l
Magnesium	0.7–1.0 mmol/l
Phosphate	0.7–1.25 mmol/l

Cholesterol	3.0–6.5 mmol/l
Protein (tot)	62–80 gm/l
Albumen	35–50 gm/l
Osmolality	275–295 mosm/kg
Bilirubin	3–17 umol/l
Thyroxine	60–160 nmol/l
Free T3	3.0–8.6 pmol/l

Enzymes

AST	5–15 u/l
HBD	50–150 u/l
GGT	5–37 u/l
CPK	less than 50 u/l
Alk. phos	100–280 u/l

Blood clotting

Prothrombin time	14–17 s
Kaolin partial thromboplastin time	35–42 s
Thrombin time	12–15 s

Normal values in urine

Amino acid nitrogen	3.6–21 mmol/l
Calcium	2.5–7.5 mmol/l
Chloride	170–250 mmol/l
Creatinine	9–17 mmol/l
Creatinine clearance	80–110 ml/min
Osmolality	40–1400 mosm/kg
Potassium	40–120 mmol/l
Sodium	100–250 mmol/l
Urea	170–600 mmol/l

Drug levels in blood

Atenolol	0.1–1.0 mg/l
Amiodarone	0.6–2.5 mg/l
Desethylamiodarone	0.6–2.5 mg/l
Digoxin levels	1.5–2.5 μg/l
	Toxicity likely if greater than 3.5μg/l
Disopyramide	2.0–5.0 mg/l
Flecainide	0.4–1.0 mg/l
Lignocaine	2.0–5.0 mg/l
Metoprolol	0.05–0.4 mg/l
Mexilitene	0.8–2.0 mg/l
Propranol	50–100 μg/l
Tocainide	3.5–9.0 mg/l

Verapamil	0.1–0.2 mg/l
Norverapamil	0.1–0.2 mg/l
Vancomycin levels	Pre less than 10, post less than 50
Gentamicin levels	Pre less than 2, post less than 6
	Both post levels 10 mins after i.v. dose

Blood gas conversion table

				mm Hg		
0	30	40	60	90	100	120
0	4	5.2	8	12	13.3	16
					KPa	
0	15		30	45		60
0	2		4	6		8
60	75		90	105		120
8	10		12	14		16
120	135		150	165		180
16	18		20	22		24

(mm Hg × 0.133 = KPa)
(KPa × 7.519 = mm Hg)

Oxygen delivery = Hb × arterial saturat'n × cardiac output × 13.4
N.R. 800–1000 ml/min

Oxygen uptake = Hb × (art-venous) sat'n × cardiac output × 13.4
N.R. 200–240 ml/min

Pacemaker code

Position in code	Meaning	Abbreviations
I	Chamber(s) paced	V. Ventricle A. Atrium D. Double
II	Chamber(s) sensed	V. Ventricle A. Atrium D. Double O. None
III	Mode of response	T. Trigger I. Inhibit D. Double O. None R. Reverse
IV	Programmable functions	P. Programmable Rate and/or output M. Multiprogrammable
V	Special tachyarrhythmia functions	B. Burst N. Normal rate competition S. Scanning E. External

20
Useful drugs

Drugs are to be administered intravenously unless otherwise stated.

Acyclovir   200 mg 5/day p.o.
Adrenaline   Bolus: 0.1–0.5 mg. Infusion: 1.5 μg/min
                         upwards
Amiloride   5–10 mg p.o.
Aminophylline   Bolus: 125–250 mg. Infusion: 0.5 mg/kg/h
Amiodarone   3 mg/kg loading then 900 mg to give a total of
                         1200 mg in first 24 hours
                         600 mg in next 24 hours
Anistreplase   30 units slow i.v. bolus
(APSAC)
Aspirin   75 mg alternate days or 300 mg o.d. as anti-
                         platelet medication
                         600 mg PR for pyrexia
Atenolol   50–100 mg p.o.
Atropine   Bolus: 0.4–1.2 mg
Azathioprine   2–3 mg/kg/day (monitor WBC)
Benzyl   600 mg 6 hourly
penicillin
Bretyllium   Bolus: 100–250 mg. Infusion: 0.5 mg/min
Bumetamide   Bolus: 0.25–5 mg
Calcium Cl   Bolus: 5–10 mmol
Captopril   6.25 mg test dose then start at 6.25 mg t.d.s
                         p.o.
Cefotaxime   1–2 g t.d.s.
Cephradine   500 mg 6 hourly
Chlormethiazole   1–4 ml/min (0.8% solution)
infusion
Chlorpheniramine   Bolus 10 mg
Chlorpromazine   Bolus 5–10 mg

Cyclosporin	2–4 mg/kg according to blood levels (usually p.o.)
Diazepam	Bolus: 5–10 mg
Digoxin	0.062–0.5 mg
	Digitalising dose; 0.75 mg/m^2 surface area
Diltiazem	60 mg t.d.s. p.o.
Dipyridamole	100 mg 8 hourly p.o.
Disopyramide	Bolus: 100 mg Infusion; 0.4 mg/kg/h
Dobutamine	5–20 μg/kg/min
Dopamine	2–5 μg/kg/min (renal); 5–10 ug/kg/min (cardiac)
Doxapram	1 to 1.5 mg/kg bolus, then 0.5 to 4 mg/min (according to response)
Enalapril	2.5–5 mg test dose, then build up to 10–20 mg (usually) o.d. p.o.
Enoximone	*Initial therapy*
	Either 0.5 to 1.0 mg/kg slowly, further doses of 0.5 mg/kg every 30 min until a response is obtained or a total initial dose of 3.0 mg/kg is reached or infusion at a rate of 90 μg/kg/min for 10–30 min until the required response is achieved.
	Maintenance therapy
	Either repeat initial dose (not more than 3.0 mg/kg) every 3–6 hours
	or infusion at a rate of 5–20 μg/kg/min.
Erythromycin	500 mg 6 hourly
Ethacrynic acid	Bolus 25–50 mg
Flecainide	2 mg/kg over 10–30 min (max 150 mg)
	Infusion start at 1.5 mg/kg/h for 1 hour decreased to 0.25 mg/kg/h oral; 100–400 mg/day
Flucloxacillin	500 mg 6 hourly
Flumazenil	0.2 mg repeated to maximum of 1 mg
Frusemide	From 10 mg to 500 mg according to circumstances
Ganciclovir	5 mg/kg over one hour twice daily for 14–21 days (2.5 mg/kg if creatinine is greater than 200 μmol/l)
Gentamicin	1 mg/kg 8 hourly (check levels)
Glyceryl tri-nitrate	0.5 mg s/l Infusion 0.5 to 10 μg/kg/min Bolus 0.5–1 mg slow i.v.
Haloperidol	Bolus 2–10 mg
Heparin	5000 u s.c. 8 hourly
	8000 u i.v. then 750–1250 u/h by infusion (DVT or PE)
	25 000 u i.v. before bypass
Insulin	Sliding scale; 60 u actrapid in 60 ml/N/saline at 0–10 ml/h to keep BM stix at 10–14 mmol/l

Isoprenaline	Bolus 0.2–0.5 mg; infusion 1.5 μg/min upwards
Isosorbide DN	Infusion 2–10 mg/h
Labetalol	10 mg increments to 50 mg slow i.v.
	Infusion up to 2 mg/min
Lignocaine	Bolus 50–100 mg. Infusion 1–4 mg/min
Mannitol	Bolus 10–20 g (50–100 ml of 20% solution)
Metaraminol	Bolus 0.5–2.5 mg
Methoxamine	Bolus 1–5 mg
Methyl prednisolone	250–1000 mg according to use
Metoclopramide	Bolus 10 mg
Metoprolol	Up to 5 mg over 5 min up to 300 mg/day p.o.
Mexilitene	Bolus 100–250 mg. Infusion 0.5 mg/min
Midazolam	Bolus 1–5 mg. Infusion 1–5 mg/h
Naloxone	Bolus 0.8–2 mg repeated as necessary
Nifedipine	5–20 mg s.l. or p.o.
Noradrenaline	Bolus 0.05–0.1 mg; infusion 1.5 μg/min upwards
Pancuronium	Bolus 6–8 mg repeated at 2–4 mg
Papaveretum	Bolus 2.5–5 mg i.v.
	10–20 mg i.m.
	Infusion 1–6 mg/h
Paracetamol	500–1000 mg p.o. or p.r.
Pethidine	Bolus 0.025–0.75 mg i.v.
	0.5–1 mg i.m.
	Infusion 5–15 mg/h
Phentolamine	Bolus 5–10 mg
Phenylephrine	Bolus 0.2–1 mg
Practolol	Bolus 1–5 mg slowly
Prochlorperazine	Bolus 12.5 mg
Propranolol	Bolus 1–5 mg slowly
Prostacyclin	1–10 nanograms/kg/min
	Titrate according to response.
	Monitor blood pressure with care.
Protamine	25–50 mg increments slowly after reversal of heparinization. Reversal dosage depends on ACT
Quinidine	300–600 mg 6 hourly p.o.
Ranitidine	50 mg 8 hourly i.v. 150 mg 12 hourly p.o.
Salbutamol	Bolus 250 μg slowly. Infusion 2.5–20 μg/min
Sodium nitroprusside	Infusion 0.5–10 μg/kg/min
Streptokinase	Infusion 500 000 u over 12 h then 100 000 u/h give chlorpheniramine 10 mg i.v. before
Sucralfate	1 g t.d.s. p.o.
Suxamethonium	Bolus 20–100 mg
Temazepam	10–20 mg p.o.
TPA	Tissue plasminogen activator; 1.5 mg/kg to a maximum of 100 mg
	10% over 2 minutes

	50% over next 1 hour
	40% over next hour
Tranexamic acid	1 g t.d.s.
Vecuronium	Bolus 80–100 µg/kg; infusion 50–80 µg/kg/h
Verapamil	Bolus 2.5–10 mg slowly
	Infusion of 2–20 mg/h

21
Drug infusion charts

Weight	75 kg	Drug	Dopamine
Concentration	200 mg		
	100 ml	2000	μg/ml
		26.67	μg/kg/ml
		0.44	μg/kg/min at 1 ml/h

rate ml/h	μg/kg/min	rate ml/h	μg/kg/min
1	0.44	13	5.72
2	0.88	14	6.16
3	1.32	15	6.60
4	1.76	16	7.04
5	2.20	17	7.48
6	2.64	18	7.92
7	3.08	19	8.36
8	3.52	20	8.80
9	3.96	25	11.00
10	4.40	30	13.20
11	4.84	35	15.40
12	5.28	40	17.60

Weight	75 kg	Drug	Dobutamine
Concentration	250 mg		
	100 ml	2500	μg/ml
		33.33	μg/kg/ml
		0.56	μg/kg/min at 1 ml/h

rate ml/h	μg/kg/min	rate ml/h	μg/kg/min
1	0.56	13	7.28
2	1.12	14	7.84
3	1.68	15	8.40
4	2.24	16	8.96
5	2.80	17	9.52
6	3.36	18	10.08
7	3.92	19	10.64
8	4.48	20	11.20
9	5.04	25	14.00
10	5.60	30	16.80
11	6.16	35	19.60
12	6.72	40	22.40

Weight	75 kg	Drug	Adrenaline
Concentration	1 mg		Isoprenaline
	100 ml		Noradrenaline
		10	μg/ml
		0.1625	μg/min at 1 ml/h

rate ml/h	μg/min	rate ml/h	μg/kg/min
1	0.16	13	2.12
2	0.33	14	2.28
3	0.49	15	2.44
4	0.65	16	2.60
5	0.81	17	2.77
6	0.98	18	2.93
7	1.14	19	3.09
8	1.30	20	3.26
9	1.46	25	4.07
10	1.63	30	4.88
11	1.79	35	5.70
12	1.95	40	6.51

Weight	75 kg	Drug	Lignocaine
Concentration	1000 mg		
	100 ml	10 000	µg/ml
		133.33	µg/kg/ml
		2.22217	µg/kg/min at 1 ml/min
		166.66275	µg/min at 1 ml/h

rate ml/h	µg/kg/min	µg/min	rate ml/h	µg/kg/min	µg/min
1	2.222	166.66	13	28.89	2166.62
2	4.444	333.33	14	31.11	2333.28
3	6.667	499.99	15	33.33	2499.94
4	8.889	666.65	16	35.56	2666.60
5	11.11	833.31	17	37.78	2833.27
6	13.33	999.98	18	40.00	2999.93
7	15.56	1166.64	19	42.22	3166.59
8	17.78	1333.30	20	44.44	3333.26
9	20.00	1499.96	25	55.55	4166.57
10	22.22	1666.63	30	66.67	4999.88
11	24.44	1833.29	35	77.78	5833.20
12	26.67	1999.95	40	88.89	6666.51

For this table there are conversion factors;

(1) For different body weight × 75/new weight
(2) For different drug dose × new dose/1000
(3) For different volume × 100/new volume

There is an alternative way of making up infusions; make up (6 × body weight) mg/100 ml, then the infusion rate in ml/h equals the infusion rate in µg/kg/min

Further reading

Regional and Applied
R. J. Last
(7th edn.) Churchill Livingstone
1984

Gray's Anatomy
P. L. Williams and R. Warwick
(36th edn.) Churchill Livingstone
1980

*Best and Taylor's Physiological Basis of Medical
Practice*
J. B. West (ed.)
(11th edn.) Williams and Wilkins
1985

Review of Medical Physiology
W. F. Ganong
(11th edn.) Lange Medical Publications
1983

Clinical Pharmacology
D. R. Laurence
Churchill Livingstone

Goodman and Gillman's the Pharmacological Basis of Therapeutics
A. G. Gilman, L. S. Goodman, T. W. Rall and F. Murad
(7th edn.) Macmillan Publishing Company
1985

Gibbon's Surgery of the Chest
D. C. Sabiston and F. C. Spencer
(4th edn.) W. B. Saunders
1983

Cardiac Surgery
J. W. Kirklin and B. G. Barratt-Boyes
John Wiley and Sons
1986

Surgery of Coronary Artery Disease
D. J. Wheatley (ed.)
Chapman and Hall
1986

Towards Safer Cardiac Surgery
D. B. Longmore (ed.)
MTP Press Ltd
1981

*McGoon's Cardiac Surgery:
an Interprofessional Approach to Patient Care*
K. M. McCauley, A. N. Brest and D. C. McGoon
F. A. Davis Company
1985

An Atlas of Cardiology
N. Conway
Wolfe Medical Publications
1977

Infection in Cardiothoracic Intensive Care
R. Freeman and F. K. Gould
Edward Arnold
1988

Intensive Care Manual
T. E. Oh
(2nd edn.) Butterworths
1987

Name	Telephone Number	Bleep Number

Intensive care unit
Theatres
Anaesthetic office
Perfusionists office
Blood bank
Haematology
Coagulation
Surgical ward
Surgical ward
Cardiology ward
Cardiology ward
Coronary care unit
Catheter laboratory
Radiology
Secretaries
Other

Index